Comfort Touch®

Massage for the Elderly and the Ill

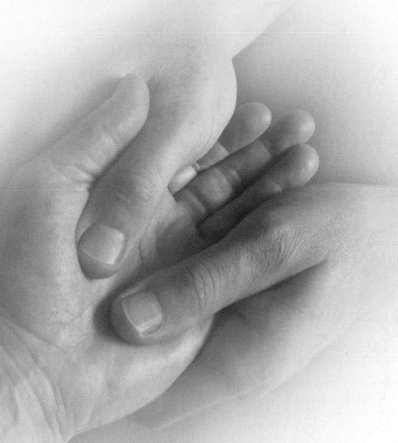

Mary Kathleen Rose, BA, LMT

Wolters Kluwer | Lippincott Williams & Wilkins
Health

Philadelphia · Baltimore · New York · London
Buenos Aires · Hong Kong · Sydney · Tokyo

Acquisitions Editor: John Goucher
Managing Editor: Linda G. Francis
Marketing Manager: Zhan Caplan
Senior Production Editor: Debra Schiff
Creative Director: Doug Smock
Compositor: Circle Graphics

Cover photo by Ian Frechette. Figure 1-1 by Stuart Ryan. Figures 1-2 and 2-4 used by permission of Nina Hart. Figure 3-1 used by permission of HospiceCare of Boulder and Broomfield Counties. Figures 3-5, 3-8, 3-9, 4-1, 4-8, 4-9 by Evelyn Funderburk. Figure 6-8 by Theresa Dent and Figure 9-7 by Fred Schulerud. All other photos by author.

9 8 7 6 5 4 3 2 1

Library of Congress Cataloging-in-Publication Data

Rose, Mary Kathleen.
   Comfort touch : massage for the elderly and the ill / Mary Kathleen Rose.
       p. ; cm.
   Includes bibliographical references and index.
   ISBN 978-0-7817-9829-7
   1. Massage therapy. 2. Touch—Therapeutic use. 3. Older people—Care. 4. Palliative treatment.
   5. Terminal care. I. Title.
   [DNLM: 1. Massage. 2. Empathy. 3. Touch. WB 537 R7978c 2010]
   RM721.R82 2010
   615.8'22—dc22

2008030647

To purchase additional copies of this book, call our customer service department at **(800) 638-3030** or fax orders to **(301) 223-2320**. International customers should call **(301) 223-2300**.

Visit Lippincott Williams & Wilkins on the Internet: http://www.lww.com. Lippincott Williams & Wilkins customer service representatives are available from 8:30 am to 6:00 pm, EST.

For Fred V. Schulerud

*Thank you for all your love and support,
your comforting touch, and for
keeping the refrigerator stocked while
I wrote this book. The simple acts
of love are the most important.*

*C*omfort Touch: Massage for the Elderly and the Ill is a textbook designed to inform the caregiver who is interested in bringing the benefits of touch to a broad range of people in need. It will give the reader the confidence to practice massage in a variety of settings, including hospices, hospitals, skilled nursing facilities, and home care. The practitioner can learn techniques that are safe and appropriate for the population for whom conventional massage may cause discomfort or even injury. It is a resource whose time has come after many years of practice, exploration, and refinement. It gives the reader an understanding of the physical and emotional needs of the elderly and those suffering from chronic illness and/or injury.

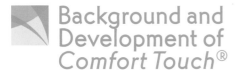

Background and Development of Comfort Touch®

The specific modality of Comfort Touch developed from my work as a massage therapist with HospiceCare of Boulder and Broomfield Counties in Colorado, which began in 1989. Building on my private practice, which included elderly clients and those with chronic illnesses, I adapted techniques derived or influenced by shiatsu, acupressure, integrative massage, and body energy therapies. With input from other massage therapists who worked with hospice, as well as the feedback of hospice staff and caregivers, I developed a training program for those interested in offering massage to patients and their families. Since 1991—in workshops, classes, and in-services held across the United States—thousands of people, including massage therapists and other healthcare professionals (nurses, nursing assistants, physical and occupational therapists), as well as family caregivers, have been introduced to the basic principles and techniques of Comfort Touch.

The guiding principles of Comfort Touch can be summarized by the acronym SCRIBE, which stands for *Slow, Comforting, Respectful, Into Center, Broad,* and *Encompassing.* These words serve as a reminder to the

practitioner of Comfort Touch regarding the rhythm, intention, attitudes, and techniques of this modality. Understanding of these principles guides the practitioner in creating a nurturing experience for the client.

Audience

This book is written with the following people in mind:

- **Massage practitioners:** Practicing massage therapists who are interested in working with the elderly and the ill will find this information a useful source of continuing education to broaden their base of practice. Adherence to the concepts presented and use of the techniques illustrated will also serve to enhance the quality of overall effectiveness in their general practice of massage.
- **Massage therapy students:** When introduced as a part of the core curriculum and training in massage therapy, the principles and techniques of Comfort Touch provide a starting place in massage therapy education, allowing students versatility from the beginning of their training.
- **Nursing and allied health professionals:** The information herein provides a valuable complement for health professionals in the fields of medicine, nursing, physical therapy, and occupational therapy. Many have used these concepts and techniques to enhance the effectiveness of the work they do. For example, a few minutes of Comfort Touch practiced on a patient about to undergo a medical procedure can have a calming effect. Use of techniques that are soothing to the patient helps to foster trust in the medical practitioner, thereby contributing to greater patient satisfaction and compliance with treatment plans.

Organization of Content

The first two chapters of the book give necessary background information, leading to the connection with the client in Chapter 3. The fourth and fifth chapters detail the guiding principles and techniques of *Comfort Touch*. The later chapters provide supporting information for the individual offering massage in a medical setting.

Special Features

- Photographs and illustrations are used throughout to clarify the text and demonstrate the techniques.
- Stories and examples relating to the use of Comfort Touch are included to inspire the reader with the range of possibilities for both the givers and receivers of touch.
- "Hints for Practice" boxes provide important information about the practical application of the content.
- Chapter Summaries highlight the most salient points in each chapter.
- Questions for review are intended to guide the reader toward greater personal awareness and professional growth.
- A glossary of key terms provides definitions of words or phrases that may be unfamiliar to the reader, or of familiar terms that are used in a unique context.
- An annotated bibliography details useful resources to support the practitioner of *Comfort Touch*.

How to Use

Although comprehensive in the material presented, this book is not intended to replace the need for professional-level training and/or supervision. Ideally, it can be used as part of a course on massage in the medical setting. It can be useful to anyone who has the necessary interest and passion to bring comfort to the people most in need of touch. By contributing to the understanding of the physical and psycho-emotional aspects of aging and illness, this text can foster a greater sense of compassion in those who work in a healthcare system.

Read this book with pencil or marker in hand, underlining the words as they speak to you. Make your own notes and comments in the margin. Study the material with other students, giving each other feedback as you learn and practice new skills. Enjoy the journey of discovery opening to you as you share the gift of touch with the elderly, the ill, or anyone in need of a caring touch.

Additional Resources

Comfort Touch: Massage for the Elderly and the Ill includes additional resources for both instructors and students that are available on the book's companion website at thePoint.lww.com/Rose.

Instructors

Approved adopting instructors will be given access to the following additional resources:

- 6-Hour Syllabus
- 16-Hour Syllabus

Students

Students who have purchased *Comfort Touch: Massage for the Elderly and the Ill* have access to the following additional resources:

- Video clips
- CARE notes with and without pain scales
- Intake forms
- Articles and reports

In addition, purchasers of the text can access the searchable Full Text online by going to the *Comfort Touch: Massage for the Elderly and the Ill* website at thePoint.lww.com/Rose. See the inside front cover of this text for more details, including the passcode you will need to gain access to the website.

Acknowledgments

My heartfelt thanks to the many people who contributed to the creation of this book:

Ian Frechette, my son, technical guru, webmaster, and thoughtful advisor. My deepest gratitude for your many hours of expert assistance on this project over the years, and a special thank you for your work in creating the beautiful photograph on the cover.

Mary Ann Foster—for your unending personal and professional support and encouragement. Thanks for making me laugh and reminding me that life is too serious to always take so seriously.

Bret Williamson—for your personal friendship and assistance in teaching over the years. Thank you for your insistence that I write the original outline for this book in 2000.

The editorial and production team at Lippincott Williams & Wilkins—with appreciation to Pete Darcy for believing in this project from the beginning; to Carol Loyd for making me a better writer; and with special gratitude to Linda Francis for your wisdom, and your thoughtful, consistent and compassionate guidance in this process.

HospiceCare of Boulder and Broomfield Counties—for the support of the administrative and clinical staffs in the development of the Comfort Touch program. Many thanks to all the massage therapists and Comfort Touch volunteers who have so generously offered of their time and talents to bring the benefits of touch to hundreds of patients and their families over the years.

Boulder College of Massage Therapy—many thanks to all the students who have participated in the hospice internship program since 1995, and shared your heartfelt stories with me of the joys and challenges of working with people in the most vulnerable times of their lives.

Morgan Community College, Department of Health Professions—many thanks to all the students in my massage classes from 1997–2002, who took Comfort Touch into numerous clinical settings. Your commitment and spirit of adventure continues to inspire me.

Many thanks to those pioneering individuals who have shared their vision of massage for the elderly and the ill and for those in medical settings with me, including: Karen Gibson, Irene Smith, Dawn Nelson, the late Cynthia Myers, Patrick Davis, and the late Dietrich Miesler. A very special thank you to Gayle MacDonald for recommending me to LWW to write this book.

Deepest thanks to the following people for creating opportunities for me to share the work of Comfort Touch with health professionals across the country: Lois Postlewaite and Shirley Sell of HEALTH EDucation Network; Leslie A. Young and Darren Buford, editors extraordinaire; Susun S. Weed, my mentor and friend; and Terry Chase and the entire research team at Craig Hospital.

My unending appreciation to all of the people and their families who allowed me to enter their lives and photograph them in the most tender moments in every phase of life. Your spirits shine through and touch all who hold this book in their hands.

Reviewers

Laura Allen, BA, MS, NCMBT
Thera-ssage
Rutherfordton, North Carolina

Lorraine Berté, RN, LMT
Downeast School of Massage
Brunswick, Maine

Karen Casciato, LMT
Portland, Oregon

Mary Duquin, PhD
Associate Professor
Department of Health and Physical Activity
University of Pittsburgh
Pittsburgh, Pennsylvania

Mary Ann Foster, BA, CMT
Boulder College of Massage Therapy
Boulder, Colorado

Contents

Introduction to Comfort Touch

> Only the touch can tell it true
> That I am human and close to you.
> —Anne U. White

*C*omfort Touch is an approach to massage that gives special consideration to the physical and emotional needs of the elderly and the ill. Its primary intention is to provide comfort through techniques that promote deep relaxation and relief from pain. As the practice of therapeutic massage develops in prevalence among the general population, interest grows in extending the benefits of touch to those for whom conventional massage can cause discomfort or even injury. The techniques of Comfort Touch can be safely practiced by massage therapists and other healthcare providers in a variety of settings, including hospices, hospitals, long-term care facilities, and home care. Adherence to the concepts presented will also serve to enhance the quality of overall effectiveness in the general practice of therapeutic massage.

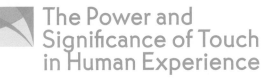

The Power and Significance of Touch in Human Experience

A human baby must be touched to survive. Even before it begins to take nourishment via the mouth and digestive system, it is comforted and nourished by touch. The mother of a newborn instinctively draws her baby to her, embracing it, providing warmth and safety (Figure 1-1).

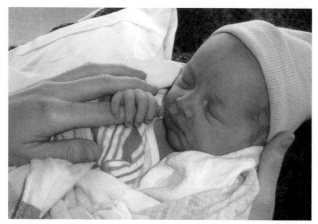

FIGURE 1-1. Mother and baby. Touch is mutually comforting for a mother and her newborn infant.

The sense of touch is the oldest of the senses. Through the skin the newborn learns about its environment. Even as the other senses—taste, hearing, sight, and smell—develop, touch remains a significant means of communication with the world surrounding the growing child. At the end of life, the process reverses as the individual's abilities to see, hear, and taste diminish. The sense of touch, however, remains as a primary means of connection and communication with the surrounding world (Figure 1-2).

Human beings experience the sense of touch in many ways throughout the course of a lifetime. The sensations and perceptions of the tactile system contribute to the rich diversity of human experience as it informs us about the objects and people in our environment. We are nurtured through touch. Touch is a means of showing care and affection. Touch is an integral part of sports and play. Touch is a means of exerting power and control. Touch is used to assess and diagnose illness, and to assist in healing.

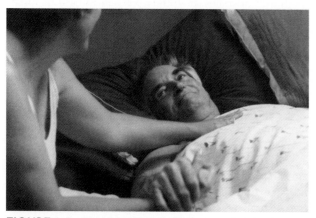

FIGURE 1-2. Hospice patient. Woman comforts her husband near the end of his life.

Attitudes and values concerning touch vary among people of different social, cultural, and religious backgrounds. The expression and experiences of touch within the family shape other relationships as a child matures into an adult. Experiences within the social network of extended family and peer groups further shape the individual's attitudes regarding touch. The sense of touch can bring about both the experiences of pleasure as well as of pain or suffering.

Touch and Sensation

To understand more about the range of the human experience and the sense of touch, it is helpful to understand how touch is felt and perceived by an individual. **Sensation** is a physical feeling derived from input to specialized receptors and sense organs of the nervous system that respond to stimuli or changes in the environment and convert the input into a nerve impulse. The impulse is conducted along a nerve pathway to the brain. A region of the brain translates the impulse into a sensation.

The skin is replete with a rich network of nerve endings and specialized tactile receptors that allow a person to experience pain, pressure, vibration, and temperature (Figure 1-3).

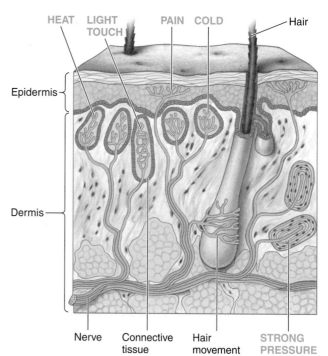

FIGURE 1-3. Tactile receptors in the skin. Specialized receptors for pain, heat and cold, light, and strong pressure are located throughout the skin. Impulses to these receptors are conducted via a nerve pathway to the brain where this input is translated into sensation.

The receptors for pain, called **nociceptors**, are the most abundant and are located throughout the body.

Perception and Memory

Perception refers to the conscious registration of a sensory stimulus. While the sense of touch provides the points of access to the world around us, perception involves complex processes and engages whole body systems, including the brain and nervous system, the endocrine system, and the neurochemical reactions within those systems. Information provided through the sense of touch is important for the safety of the organism. For example, the perception of pain may result in a response that causes one to pull back from the source of injury, such as extreme heat or pressure, that could cause tissue damage.

Memories present in the nervous system, and the ways in which they are interpreted by the brain, contribute to the perception of information received by the tactile receptors. A person's expectations and receptivity to touch influence how that touch is perceived. Memories of past pleasures and/or pain and trauma contribute to a person's current perception. Input through the other senses of sight and hearing also contribute to the perception of touch. For example, soothing words which accompany touch give added meaning to the tactile sensation.

Learning is a process of adapting to new information. Perceptions that are reinforced by subsequent experience become permanent impressions. The more a neural pathway is used in early childhood, the more it becomes **myelinated**, a process by which nerve tissue is insulated, improving electrical conductivity. This is how our basic patterns of perceiving and responding to the world are formed. These patterns—which include our preferences, tastes, fears, and ways of relating to the outside world—are largely formed in childhood. Change is possible in later years by myelinating new pathways, but the initial circuitry remains.

When one person touches another, she or he is accessing the nervous system and memory of that person, affecting it by the input the touch is providing. This new input can reinforce old perceptions, or it can create new perceptions and memories. For example, when a patient in the hospital is touched in a comforting manner, this experience may evoke memories of the nurturing touch she or he received from a parent in childhood. In another example, the comforting touch can help to counteract the negative associations a hospitalized patient has with painful medical procedures. This new input brings the possibilities for a change in the patient's perceptions and sense of well-being.

Stimulus to the nervous system is also known to affect a range of chemical responses in the body. Touch can effect the release of natural chemicals in the body which affect the perception of pleasure or pain. For example, touch can stimulate the production of **endorphins**, which are the body's natural painkillers. Touch can also stimulate the production of **oxytocin,** a hormone associated with feelings of bonding and connection. Conversely, a painful stimulus can produce the release of **epinephrine** from the adrenal gland, which is associated with distress, fear, and anxiety.

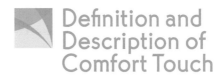

Definition and Description of Comfort Touch

Comfort Touch is a nurturing style of massage designed to be safe, appropriate, and effective for the elderly and the ill. It is adaptable to the needs of the client, and may be practiced on the person who is seated in a wheelchair, a regular chair, a recliner, a hospital bed, or a bed in the home. The technique does *not* require the use of lotions or oils, and the client may remain fully clothed.

Principles of Comfort Touch—SCRIBE

The Comfort Touch method of massage can be described by six guiding principles that can be summarized by the acronym SCRIBE, which stands for *Slow, Comforting, Respectful, Into Center, Broad,* and *Encompassing.* These words serve as a reminder to the practitioner of Comfort Touch regarding the rhythm, intention, attitudes, and techniques of this modality of massage.

The rhythm of the work is *slow;* the intention is to be *comforting* while maintaining a *respectful* attitude toward the client. Pressure is applied perpendicularly *into the center* of the part of the body being touched. Comfort Touch techniques generally rely on *broad,* full-hand contact *encompassing* the part of the body being touched. Specific attention is given to the appropriate amount of pressure to ensure a sensation that is calming and soothing. (These principles are further discussed in Chapter 4.)

Techniques of Comfort Touch

The specific techniques used in the practice of Comfort Touch are derived in large part from the Asian bodywork modalities of **Shiatsu** and **acupressure**, with influences from **Integrative Massage** and **body energy therapies.** With respect for an understanding of anatomy, as well as the Asian theories of meridians as pathways of energy in the body, Comfort Touch provides a nurturing form of contact that is safe for the individual. It satisfies the need to be touched gently, yet firmly and deliberately.

The techniques of Swedish massage, which form the basis of most massage school curriculums, may be contraindicated for people of advanced age and those affected by illness or specific physical or emotional sensitivity. For example, effleurage (gliding), petrissage (kneading), and tapotement (percussion) can cause tearing of the skin or bruising of delicate tissues. While derived from acupressure, Comfort Touch does *not* use deep thumb or finger pressure that could be painful or uncomfortable to the client.

From Integrative Massage, Comfort Touch derives the slow, nurturing rhythm of the touch, along with the emphasis on acknowledgement of the wholeness of the individual. Various body energy therapies (eg, Therapeutic Touch, Attunement, Reiki, Polarity Therapy) support the understanding and awareness of subtle energies in the body, and the importance of creating a healing environment for the client through respectful attitude and intention.

Comfort Touch is *not* "light touch" or "noncontact" touch. It is specific and consistent in application to allow the deepest relaxation and the greatest benefit to the recipient. Noncontact modalities of healing can have benefit for the patient, and these will be addressed further in Chapter 5.

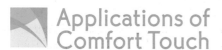

Applications of Comfort Touch

Comfort Touch is a modality of massage that can be used for a broad range of people in a variety of settings. Its emphasis on comfort makes it a useful complement to medical care, as well as a primary measure to ease the discomfort of physical and emotional pain. For the elderly and the chronically and terminally ill, the use of Comfort Touch is consistent with the philosophy of **palliative** care. Palliation refers to the inten-

tion to alleviate symptoms without the emphasis to cure the underlying disease or injury. It may involve pain management through appropriate use of drugs, as well as using other treatments and services that enhance the quality of life for the individual. Emphasis is on the care of the patients' physical, psychological, social, and spiritual comfort and well-being in an atmosphere of respect and compassion (Figure 1-4).

Who Can Benefit from Comfort Touch?

- **The elderly.** The special needs of the elderly are determined by the loss of function and the associated physiological changes of the natural aging process.
- **The chronically physically ill.** This category includes those who are suffering from, but not limited to, any of the following conditions and illnesses: heart disease, cancer, stroke, diabetes, pulmonary diseases, kidney disease, multiple sclerosis, arthritis, Parkinson's disease, amyotrophic lateral sclerosis (Lou Gehrig disease), HIV/AIDS, and fibromyalgia.[1,2]
- **The terminally ill.** Comfort Touch can provide physical and emotional support for those diagnosed with terminal illness. It can be used throughout the process, and addresses the changing needs of the individual approaching death.
- **People with Alzheimer's disease and other forms of dementia.** Some may be otherwise physically robust, or may have dementia associated with physical illness (eg, vascular dementia).[3]
- **People with acute illness or injury.** Comfort Touch can bring relief to a patient suffering from an acute illness or injury, and helps to facilitate a state of well-being during the period of recovery.

Hints for Practice

Body Ease

When you practice Comfort Touch it is important to be comfortable in your own body. Just as you attend to the needs of your clients, you must pay attention to your own posture, breathing, and efficient use of body mechanics. If you feel awkward or uncomfortable in your own body, your clients may sense that and may be distracted from their own enjoyment of the touch.

Before you begin a hands-on session, take a couple of deep, full breaths. Notice that your back is straight and your shoulders are relaxed, with your elbows resting at your sides. When you are at ease in your own body, this feeling of comfort can be translated to the person you are touching, enhancing the quality of the experience for both of you. (Refer to Body Patterning for the Practitioner in Chapter 3 for more specific suggestions.)

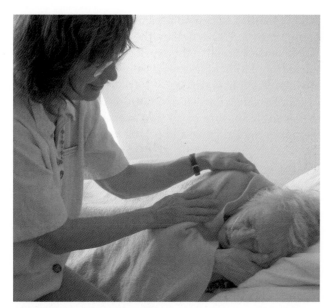

FIGURE 1-4. Palliative care. Comfort touch is a valuable component of palliative care for this elderly woman in a skilled nursing facility.

- **Pre- and postsurgical patients.** Comfort Touch can help to calm a patient before surgery. After surgery, the simple use of touch can help to alleviate pain and contribute to the healing process.
- **People with spinal cord and closed head injuries.** From the acute phase of injury to long-term rehabilitation, Comfort Touch can assist in the treatment plan, addressing issues of pain, insomnia, and emotional support.
- **Pregnant and perinatal patients.** The massage practitioner can use Comfort Touch to adapt to the changing needs of the pregnant woman and provide valuable support during labor and delivery.
- **Newborns and infants.** The simplicity and directness of this modality provide immediate comfort and stimulation to the newborn. Ongoing use of Comfort Touch techniques with the infant provides physical health benefits and emotional bonding when used by the parents or caregivers.
- **Children.** Comfort Touch is a very adaptable form of massage that is useful to share with children. Even a brief session can help to calm a child in distress, or to establish a base of meaningful communication.
- **Trauma patients and those with mental illness.** Comfort Touch has been used as a part of complementary care for those suffering from a range of mental illnesses, including anxiety, depression, bipolar disorder, eating disorders, and posttraumatic stress disorder.

- **Autistic people.** The broad, direct pressure used in Comfort Touch is calming to the over-sensitized system of the autistic child or adult.
- **Healthy people.** These principles and techniques can be applied to the general practice of massage used for wellness and stress relief.

Note that Chapter 6 contains information and specific considerations for working with these different populations. It is important to understand that there is often a greater range of functionality between individuals who have been diagnosed with a particular disease than there is between people with differing diagnoses. In this work, *we are always paying attention to the needs of the individual, rather than treating the disease itself.*

Where Is Comfort Touch Practiced?

Comfort Touch can be practiced in many settings. Many of the people who benefit from this approach to massage are unable to travel, so it is customary that the therapist works with them in their own home surroundings. Because this technique requires no special equipment, the client can be in his or her own bed, a hospital bed, a wheelchair, or a recliner. Comfort Touch is practiced in the following settings:

- **Hospitals and medical centers.** Patients may be in different areas of the facility, including pre- and postsurgical units, cardiopulmonary units, cancer treatment centers, perinatal units, etc. Permission may be required from the attending physician or other hospital staff.
- **Hospice care centers.** In-patient facilities use Comfort Touch as part of palliative care of the terminally ill.
- **Hospice home care agencies.** Home care agencies use Comfort Touch as part of palliative care of the terminally ill. These patients are living in their own homes.
- **Home health care agencies.** Home health care agencies that care for people with chronic illnesses can incorporate Comfort Touch into the ongoing care of their patients (Figure 1-5).
- **Skilled nursing and assisted-living facilities.** Residents require varying degrees of assistance from a skilled nursing staff. Massage therapists can be hired by individual residents or may contract to work with the general resident population and/or staff of the facility.
- **Retirement homes.** These homes are adapted to the needs of the elderly who are living independently. Massage therapists can be hired by individual residents.
- **Senior centers.** Usually meeting places in a community, senior centers provide gathering places

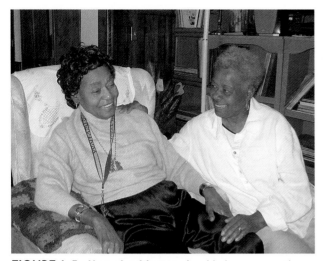

FIGURE 1-5. Home health care. An elderly woman with dementia benefits by the comforting touch of a visiting home health care nurse.

for senior men and women to enjoy meals and social, educational, and wellness programs. Massage therapy is sometimes provided in special treatment rooms at the facility.

- **Rehabilitation centers.** These facilities serve people who are recovering from injuries and/or surgery. Comfort Touch can be an adjunct therapy to physical therapy and occupational therapy.

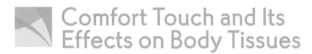

Comfort Touch and Its Effects on Body Tissues

In the elderly and the ill, there is often significant loss of muscle tone or atrophy of muscle tissue. This may be a concern for the massage therapist who is accustomed to thinking about the benefits of massage in terms of

muscle tension, and who uses techniques designed to manipulate and/or lengthen the muscles. It is important to understand that this work is not primarily about the manipulation of muscle tissue. Doing so can actually damage fragile tissue.

Rather, the practice of Comfort Touch addresses the interrelationship of all the layers of body tissues, including the structure and function of the **superficial fascia.** Composed of adipose tissue and loose connective tissue, the superficial fascia is located beneath the skin. Varying in thickness, it covers the entire body, providing insulation and protection for the deep fascia, muscles, and organs beneath it. It stores fat and water and provides passageways for nerves and blood and lymph vessels (Figure 1-6).

Skillfully applied Comfort Touch, with its emphasis on broad, encompassing pressure into the center of the body part being touched, gently warms and nurtures the superficial fascia, respecting the fluid nature of its ground substance. The radiant heat from the practitioner's hands is transferred via the fluid of the connective tissue, affecting the circulation of capillary blood and lymph. Not only is this process relaxing to the client, but it engenders a comforting feeling of warmth, ease, and fluidity in the body. The soothing warmth of human touch appeals to an individual's most primal life-affirming instincts.

Another avenue of direct sensation in the use of Comfort Touch is pressure itself. For example, when an infant is held, it is comforted by the consistency of broad, encompassing pressure. This quality of touch defines the boundaries of a safe container, and is commonly expressed as a caring touch or friendly hug between individuals to convey affection or concern. Comfort Touch is the therapeutic and skillful application of touch that respects the value and importance of this basic human need.

The body's tissues do not act independently of one another, but are part of an overall system that is affected

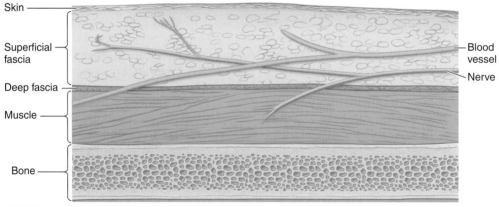

FIGURE 1-6. Tissue layers. The warmth of contact and broad pressure exerted in Comfort Touch affect the skin, superficial fascia, deep fascia, and muscle tissue.

by the input provided through touch. For example, the tension held in muscles may be released, not directly because of mechanical manipulation, but because the nerve receptors in the skin and connective tissues convey impulses to the brain, which interprets the physical contact as desirable. This engages the **parasympathetic nervous system**, eliciting a generalized relaxation response in the body.

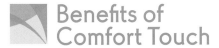

Benefits of Comfort Touch

The practice of Comfort Touch is easy to implement from a logistical standpoint, because it does not require the use of special massage tables. The practitioner works on clients in their own homes or in medical settings—wherever they are most comfortable. Also, the client does not need to disrobe, as in conventional massage. This eliminates concerns about modesty, and the logistics of undressing and draping.

Professional medical providers, family caregivers, and recipients have reported numerous benefits, both physical and psycho-emotional, of Comfort Touch as a modality.

Physical Benefits

- **Relaxation.** The recipient of Comfort Touch experiences the enjoyment and restfulness of deep relaxation. This relaxation can occur on many levels, including the physical, emotional, and mental aspects of the person.
- **Pain reduction.** Comfort Touch has a calming, sedating effect on the nervous system, decreasing the perception of pain. It offers a soothing input to the individual, helping to shift one's awareness of the pain to the awareness of pleasure, thereby interrupting the experience and perception of pain.
- **Release of general and/or specific muscle tension.** Specific techniques allow for the release of tension held in the muscles. Tension can be a result of overuse of the muscles, or it can result from the inactivity of a sedentary lifestyle.
- **Increased circulation of blood and lymph.** Massage helps to increase local circulation of blood and lymph, thereby facilitating the process of nourishing the body on a cellular level. This process can help to balance body chemistry and speed healing.
- **Increased flexibility.** Warming of the connective tissues, release of muscular tension, and improved circulation can contribute to better mobility.

- **Easier breathing.** Relaxation of the muscles and calming of the nervous system facilitate easier and deeper breathing. Specific contact pressure points in the hands and feet may help alleviate sinus congestion.
- **Improved appetite and digestion.** Clients may experience better appetite, digestion, and elimination following the mild stimulation of Comfort Touch.
- **Improved quality of sleep.** Release of tension, pain, and anxiety all contribute to better sleep.
- **Increased energy and mental alertness.** While Comfort Touch is relaxing to the body and mind, it often is energizing as well, leading to greater physical and mental alertness.

Psycho-Emotional Benefits

- **Comfort and assurance of human contact.** Touch is a way for one human being to acknowledge the importance of another. Whether in a professional or home setting, touch that is offered with kindness of intention validates this most basic of human needs.
- **Reduction of anxiety/fear/distress.** A comforting touch can bring relief from the various stresses one feels in everyday life. Often, fear and anxiety accompany physical and emotional pain, illness, and distress. Fear itself is often a cause of secondary pain or tension. This pain can lead to more fear and anxiety, which in turn lead to more pain. Comforting touch helps to break this cycle, helping the client to feel more in control of his or her own physical and emotional reality.[4]
- **Improved feelings of safety and confidence.** The consistency of contact and pressure in Comfort Touch contribute to feelings of safety and confidence. Much of the fear that accompanies illness and aging, with its pains and losses, results from the feeling of uncertainty, the fear of the unknown. Knowing what to expect, through the pleasure of touch that is predictably comfortable and nurturing, allows the recipient to relax in the moment with a feeling of confidence.
- **Relief from depression and improved feelings of self-esteem.** The gently stimulating effect of touch can lead the individual to experience a brighter outlook. Clients feel better just knowing that someone cares and is willing to be with them. Touch acknowledges their importance as human beings, contributing to feelings of trust and hope.[4]
- **Communication.** Touch is a significant and valuable way to communicate nonverbally with another person. Often it opens the door to more effective and enjoyable verbal communication as well.

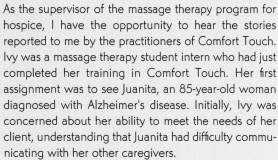

STORY

Be Simple

As the supervisor of the massage therapy program for hospice, I have the opportunity to hear the stories reported to me by the practitioners of Comfort Touch. Ivy was a massage therapy student intern who had just completed her training in Comfort Touch. Her first assignment was to see Juanita, an 85-year-old woman diagnosed with Alzheimer's disease. Initially, Ivy was concerned about her ability to meet the needs of her client, understanding that Juanita had difficulty communicating with her other caregivers.

In her initial visits Ivy used the techniques of Comfort Touch she had learned, applying broad, encompassing pressure, gently but firmly touching the patient's arms and legs while she rested in her recliner. The patient expressed her pleasure, saying, "Perfecto. You are the best." The patient relaxed with Ivy's touch, sometimes falling asleep. During one visit, she said, "You are the best of everyone who comes."

In subsequent visits Ivy felt their communication deepen, knowing that Juanita, though failing physically and mentally, would still respond to her as she was touched. Even so, Ivy still wondered at times if she could be doing more, if she was using the right combination of techniques. On one occasion, as Ivy took her frail arm to massage it, the woman said, "Be simple." Listening to this cue, Ivy responded by taking Juanita's hands and simply holding them in her own. They looked into each other's eyes. Ivy recounted that as she relaxed in her own body, continuing to hold her hands, Juanita said, "Thank you. Thank you."

"That's what I love about hospice," Ivy said to me. "I don't have to try and do anything. I just need to be present. Time passes so quickly." Ivy offered her touch with the clear intention of providing comfort, not trying to fix or change anything. From this patient, Ivy learned the wisdom of those words, "Be simple." (Figure 1-7.)

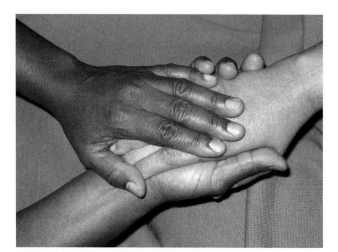

FIGURE 1-7. Hands. Holding the hand is a simple, yet powerful way to offer comfort.

  a. What is the earliest touch you remember? What are your most pleasant memories of touch as a child? As an adult?
  b. Do you have painful memories of touch as a child? As an adult?
  c. How do you learn about the world around you through your sense of touch?
  d. How do you like to be touched? By friends and family? By health professionals?
4. How do you like to be comforted? What do you do to comfort others in your life—other than touch?
5. How much of your time is spent with people who would be considered elderly or ill? What role do you play with these people?
6. In what medical settings have you spent time? In what settings or environments are you most comfortable? Where do you feel most uncomfortable?
7. What do you see as the greatest benefit of Comfort Touch? Physically? Emotionally?
8. Why are you interested in learning Comfort Touch? What do you hope to learn to benefit yourself personally and professionally?

 ## Some Questions for Getting Started

Following are some questions to ask yourself as you begin to work with Comfort Touch.

1. What is your experience in the field of medicine? As a practitioner? As a patient?
2. What is your experience in the field of massage? As a practitioner? As a client?
3. What is your own experience of touch?

Summary

- From infancy to old age, the sense of touch provides a powerful means of connection and communication to the surrounding world. It is a significant gateway to perception, memory, and relationship to others.
- Comfort Touch is a nurturing style of bodywork designed to be safe, appropriate, and effective, addressing the physical and emotional needs of the

elderly and the ill. The practitioner of Comfort Touch is guided by six principles (SCRIBE) which describe the rhythm, intention, attitudes, and techniques of this modality of massage.

- Comfort Touch provides the benefits of massage to a broad range of people including: the elderly, the chronically and terminally ill, the injured, pregnant and perinatal women, infants and children, as well as those suffering from trauma or mental illness. It is also beneficial to the general population of people who appreciate the value of nurturing touch.

- Comfort Touch can be practiced in a wide variety of settings including; hospitals, hospices, skilled-nursing facilities, and home care. The client can be in a hospital bed, a wheelchair, recliner, or her or his own bed at home.

- The practice of Comfort Touch addresses the inter-relationship of all the layers of body tissue. Rather than emphasizing manipulation of muscles, it provides the radiant warmth of contact and broad, encompassing pressure, thereby eliciting the relaxation response.

- Many physical and psycho-emotional benefits have been attributed to the practice of Comfort Touch. These include relaxation, pain reduction, increased local circulation of blood and lymph, improved quality of sleep, reduction of anxiety, and relief from depression.

Review Questions

1. Describe the significance of touch in the development of a human being. For example, how does an infant or child learn about his or her world through the sense of touch?
2. What are the functions of the tactile receptors in the skin?
3. What is the primary intention of Comfort Touch?

4. What are the six principles of Comfort Touch?
5. Who can benefit by receiving Comfort Touch? Give five examples of populations for whom Comfort Touch can be beneficial.
6. Where is Comfort Touch practiced? List four examples of settings where Comfort Touch is appropriate.
7. Briefly describe the effect of Comfort Touch on body tissues.
8. List five physical benefits of Comfort Touch.
9. List three psychosocial benefits of Comfort Touch.

References

1. Beider S. An ethical argument for integrated palliative care [monograph online]. Oxford University Press, eCAM; 2005. http://ecam.oxfordjournals.org/cgi/reprint/neh089 v1.pdf. Accessed June 2007.
2. UF pilot study shows massage, relaxation reduce sickle cell anemia pain. *University of Florida News.* September 25, 2000. http://news.ufl.edu/2000/09/25/massage/. Accessed June 2007.
3. Yang M-H, Wu S-C, Lin J-G, Lin L-C. The efficacy of acupressure for decreasing agitated behavior in dementia: a pilot study. *J Clin Nurs.* February 2007;16(2):308–315.
4. Moyer CA, Rounds J, Hannum JW. A meta-analysis of massage therapy research. *Psychol Bull.* 2004;130(1):3–18.

Suggested Reading

Aydede M. An analysis of pleasure vis-à-vis pain. *Philosophy and Phenomenological Research* [serial online]. 2000;61 (3):537–70. http://web.clas.ufl.edu/users/maydede/ pleasure.pdf. Accessed June 1, 2007.

Grant KM. Myth and musings. *Massage Today.* September 2001;1:09.

Juhan D. *Job's Body: A Handbook for Bodywork.* 3rd ed. Barry-town: Station Hill Press; 2003.

Montague A. *Touching: The Human Significance of Skin.* 3rd ed. New York: Harper & Row; 1986.

Pert C. *Molecules of Emotion: The Science Behind Body-Mind Medicine.* New York: Simon and Schuster; 1997.

Understanding Health, Illness, Loss, and Grief

> **Health is the ability to adapt to change.**
> —Anonymous

*H*ealth refers to a state of wholeness, free from physical, mental, or emotional infirmity. Derived from the same root word for *whole,* health generally describes the condition of an individual who functions optimally without evidence of disease or abnormality. But as most people age, they tend to lose the level of physical and mental ability they had when they were younger. Over time they lose function through specific disease processes, traumatic injuries, or general physiologic decline. Yet there is a wisdom and strength that comes with age and experience, often in spite of deteriorating physical and/or mental capacities. So when

referring to these special populations of the elderly and the ill, we may wonder if there is, in fact, an objective definition for what constitutes health.

 ## Concepts of Health and Disease

Throughout history and the development of modern culture, attitudes about health and disease have been diverse, changing as new information informs our understanding of the human body. For example, we take it for granted that blood circulates throughout the body via a system involving the heart, veins, and arteries. This awareness, put forth by William Harvey in the 1600s, led to the view of the body that is made up of specialized systems that work together, forming the basis of medical knowledge today. An understanding of health also includes an appreciation of the emotional and mental aspects of an individual. Mental health involves the ability to function in society with a sense of well-being, as one interacts with others through work and social relationships.

Homeostasis

The human body is composed of many systems involving a complex of functions and interactions, including movement, metabolism, sensation, circulation, immunity, respiration, reproduction, and elimination. The balanced state of all these systems and the chemical and neurological processes that control them are referred to as **homeostasis**. Change in one part of the body affects the rest of the body, allowing for constant adjustments, enabling the individual to function in the outer world, adjusting to the needs and demands of the physical and social environment. This ability to adapt to change allows the human species to thrive through a rich diversity of experience and expression.

Disease

Whereas health is the state that allows for the normal functioning of the individual, disease is experienced as the disruption of function. Disease may be **acute**, as in the case of a cold or flu, which is a temporary condition; or it may be **chronic**, as in the case of asthma or heart disease. An acute illness or injury may be totally disruptive, necessitating the temporary cessation of everyday activities. In a different way, a chronic disease will cause disruptions, but the individual can adapt, either through medical interventions and/or lifestyle changes, to continue to live a fulfilling life in spite of the illness.

Health and Wellness: Adapting to Change

For many people health is a state they take for granted. They are free from disease and able to pursue interests regarding work and social activities. For others, whose state of health is influenced by a variety of factors—including genetics, pathogens, environmental toxins, or injury—health can seem like an elusive goal, as they seek to cope with the limitations of their condition. Still others, who would generally regard themselves as healthy, ascribe to the notion of wellness in which they consciously make choices to enhance their experience of health, optimizing their mental and/or physical level of function.

The definition of health can vary from one individual to another, intricately tied to one's cultural background, social network, material resources, and personal expectations and aspirations. While we are familiar with the expression "young and healthy," it is less common to refer to someone as "old and healthy," or to talk about a "healthy diabetic." The state of health is not an objective experience. It is subjective, and ultimately refers to a person's ability to adapt to change brought about by age, life circumstance, illness, or injury.

A sense of well-being can be experienced even for the most ill or disabled person if there is sufficient support to help one adapt to her or his situation. The support offered may come from family and friends, the community, or social and medical systems, as they are available. Comfort Touch can be one of the means of assisting someone to experience a state of wellness. For many, it provides a way to affirm their inner resources and value as human beings, in spite of physical disease or debility (Figure 2-1).

Comfort Touch and Models of Medicine

Massage and bodywork as means of healing are ancient in their origins, yet have developed outside of the mainstream of modern scientific medicine. As the current

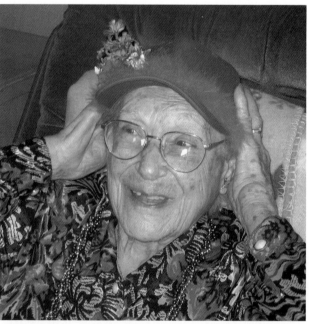

FIGURE 2-1. Enjoying life. Though living with chronic illness, this 90-year-old woman dons her hat and smiles, conveying her pleasure after receiving a session of Comfort Touch.

world of medicine expands in its understanding of the anatomy and physiology of the human body, providing ever more sophisticated treatments for disease, the general population is also looking for the value offered through alternative and complementary therapies, including therapeutic massage and bodywork. Comfort Touch, with its emphasis on safe, appropriate, and effective techniques for the elderly and the ill, provides a suitable approach to bodywork in the medical setting.

Healing versus Cure

It is crucial for the practitioners of massage and bodywork to understand the difference in intention implied by the words "healing" and "curing." **Curing** connotes the restoration of someone to a state of health, free from disease or ailment. Many resources of society are geared toward the hope of finding cures for the conditions and diseases that plague the population. Research abounds in laboratories and clinics worldwide in the quest for drugs and medical procedures to ease the suffering of patients and/or effect cures for their diseases. Great strides have been made to significantly reduce the impact of many diseases (eg, antibiotics for bacterial infections, vaccinations for contagious diseases). Surgical techniques have greatly impacted the threat of many diseases (eg, cancer, heart disease, orthopedic injuries).

Curative measures can be utilized through appropriate medical interventions, such as surgery to remove a tumor or repair a specific body part. Curing, in this sense, requires a diagnosis and an intervention by the appropriate medical personnel. The intention to cure implies a need to fix or change the circumstance of the patient. While this is appropriate, and certainly desirable when possible, this intention or attitude can be a detriment to the individual who has an incurable disease or condition.

Healing is also defined as the process of making one well or restoring to a state of health or wholeness; but, whereas curing implies the notion of ridding one of disease, healing emphasizes the acknowledgment of the individual as a whole human being, regardless of her or his current condition. The practitioner of Comfort Touch does not need to be concerned about curing someone of infirmity. Rather, the client is seen as a whole human being, in need of nourishment and care (Figure 2-2).

It is *not* the role of the massage therapist to diagnose, fix, or change the client. Rather, it is appropriate to provide the healing experience that comes by offering care that is comforting and nurturing. This allows the person to adapt to change and to feel a sense of well-being in spite of her or his condition or illness. Change

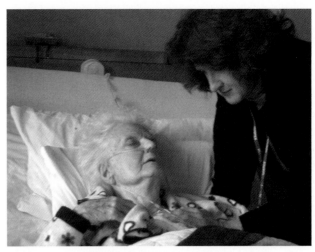

FIGURE 2-2. Hospice patient. With the caring touch provided by the Comfort Touch practitioner, this elderly woman in a hospice facility is able to rest comfortably.

can and does occur, but the emphasis is on the wholeness of the individual human being, *not* the specific disease or condition.

Definitions of Medicine

The National Institutes of Health (NIH) established the National Center for Complementary and Alternative Medicine (NCCAM) in 1998 to explore complementary and alternative healing practices (CAM), mandating research, training, and education to be made available to professionals and the public. NCCAM defines three categories of medicine:

1. **Conventional Medicine.** This form of medicine is dominant in the developed world and is practiced by holders of MD (Medical Doctor) or DO (Doctor of Osteopathy) degrees, and by allied health professionals such as physical therapists, psychologists, and registered nurses. It involves the use of diagnostic methods and technologies, standards of research or evidence-based practices, and employs the use of pharmaceutical drugs and surgical procedures.

2. **Alternative Medicine.** Defined by NCCAM, alternative medicine is used *in place of* conventional medicine. It consists of many different practices including:
   - **Biological practices.** These include the use of dietary supplements and special diets.
   - **Energy medicine.** These approaches involve practices based on an awareness of energy fields believed to surround and infuse the human body.

- **Bodywork practices.** Techniques involve manipulation or movement of the body.
- **Mind–body medicine.** Techniques are designed to enhance the mind's ability to affect bodily function and symptoms.
- **Whole medical systems.** These include systems derived from other cultural paradigms, such as the ancient systems of traditional Chinese medicine and the Ayurvedic medicine of India.

3. **Complementary Medicine.** This category includes approaches used *together with* conventional medicine, and may involve treatments included in the definition of alternative medicine. Such practices used may include: nutritional diets, energy or spiritual healing, massage, exercise, meditation, and relaxation techniques.

Comfort Touch as Complementary Medicine

Comfort Touch is a valuable complementary therapy for those being treated by conventional medicine. Based on a solid foundation and understanding of the anatomy of the body, it uses techniques which benefit the client who is undergoing medical treatment. Inherent in the intention of Comfort Touch is an appreciation of the fragility of the client, and a respect for the challenges faced by someone undergoing treatment for either acute or chronic illness. Rather than focus on contraindications to conventional massage (ie, Swedish massage), the practitioner of Comfort Touch looks at the needs of the client and finds a safe and appropriate way to offer the benefits of touch.

During a Comfort Touch session the patient remains in the position of her or his own greatest comfort. This may be in a hospital bed, regular bed, wheelchair, or recliner. This ensures the safety and comfort of the patient, and eliminates the necessity of using a massage table. The therapist adjusts her or his own body mechanics to work most easily and efficiently.

The practitioner of Comfort Touch learns to work cooperatively as part of the health care team providing services to the patient. Often she or he is in a position to offer helpful insight to other caregivers. Communication with staff is a two-way street enhancing the effectiveness of care for the patient, as changes in the patient's health status are shared between medical staff and massage therapist.

Comfort Touch as Nourishing Tradition

While Comfort Touch takes its place as a complementary therapy in the medical setting, or in practice with the elderly and the ill, it also holds merit for *any* individual in need of nurturing touch. The intention of this modality of bodywork resonates with the most basic of human experiences—the bonding that comes with human contact. The therapeutic value of Comfort Touch lies in the specific use of techniques which optimize the relaxation response, enhancing the recipient's sense of well-being.

The general principles and specific techniques of Comfort Touch can be used by anyone who wishes to provide a therapeutic experience of touch. Without the need to diagnose, fix, or change the "problems" of the client, the practitioner can focus on the true experience of healing which comes about by being truly present with another human being. From the place of deep, nurturing connection, Comfort Touch also provides a starting point for working deeper into the layers of the body's tissues (eg, the muscles and deep fascia). The broad, encompassing contact of Comfort Touch warms the tissues, allowing changes on a deep level, without the manipulative and sometimes painful processes of other approaches to bodywork.

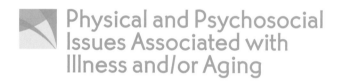

Physical and Psychosocial Issues Associated with Illness and/or Aging

Aging is a process involving growth, maturation, and change from childhood, puberty, young adulthood, through middle and late age. It involves biological changes in the body, psychological and mental development, and adaptation to life circumstances. The life span of Americans has been increasing over the past century, owing in part to decreases in infant mortality. Other factors that influence longevity are heredity, greater access to medical care, and lifestyle. More and more older people are enjoying healthy, productive lives well beyond middle age and the demands of raising a family, engaging in full-time employment, etc.

In the United States there is a growing percentage of the population over age 65, with a growing number of the population living over 85 years of age. People aged 65 and over represented 12.4% of the population in the year 2005, but are expected to grow to be 20% of the population by 2030. According to the U.S. Department of Health and Human Services' Administration on Aging, the population over the age 65 will increase from 35 million in 2000 to 40 million in 2010 (a 15% increase), and then to 55 million in 2010 (a 36% increase for that decade). The population over the age of 85 is projected to increase from 4.2 million in 2000 to 6.1 million in 2010 (a 40% increase), and then to 7.3 million in 2020 (a 44% increase for that decade).[1]

Physical Issues Associated with Aging

There are physical issues associated with aging itself, as well as physiological processes involved with a myriad of acute and chronic illnesses. Even without a specific diagnosis of disease, aging involves a process called **senescence.** This is the process by which the capacity for cell division, growth, and function is lost over time, ultimately leading to death. Along with this natural course of change, many individuals also suffer from specific acute or chronic diseases, which affect the functioning of organs and systems in the body.

Aging itself is not a disease, but any of the following changes can be observed in the older person. Note that individuals of any age vary tremendously from one another in their physical condition.

- **Skin and Connective Tissue.** Loss of elasticity; decrease in lubricating secretions; skin may be dry and itchy; small capillaries increase in fragility, leading to greater vulnerability to bruising; full hydration of skin may become more difficult.
- **Muscular/Skeletal System.** Changes in bone density (osteoporosis); stiffness or pain in joints (arthritis); reduced elasticity and flexibility of tendons and ligaments; weakness or spasm in muscles; decreased range of motion.
- **Cardiovascular System.** Weakness or changes in the heart muscle; decreased elasticity of blood vessels, changes in thickness of blood vessels (arteriosclerosis); changes in blood pressure; impaired circulation of blood and lymph, particularly to the extremities.
- **Respiratory System.** Decline in lung capacity and effectiveness of breathing.
- **Immune System.** Decline in resistance to infection.
- **Gastrointestinal System.** Decrease in motility and rate or effectiveness of digestion and elimination; decrease in production of digestive juices, increase in insulin resistance; changes in appetite.
- **Genitourinary System.** Decrease in muscle tone of bladder and muscles controlling urination; enlargement of prostate gland in males; changes in genital tissue and functions.
- **Endocrine System.** Changes in secretions of endocrine glands affecting many systems in the body (eg, thyroid hormone, insulin, sex hormones).
- **Neurologic System.** Changes in mental function, memory, or cognition; loss of fine motor control; changes in patterns of sleep.

Other physical issues associated with aging involve changing levels of function with the special senses.

These changes affect the way people experience the world around them. Here are some examples:

- **Vision.** Changes in elasticity of the eye, affecting vision; increased sensitivity to light; other changes affecting vision (eg, cataracts, glaucoma, macular degeneration).
- **Hearing.** Gradual loss of hearing or sensitivity to pitch and background noises; slower processing of auditory information.
- **Taste and Smell.** Decline in number of taste buds and deterioration of the sense of smell; loss of appetite.
- **Touch.** Increased or decreased sensitivity to touch.

Physical Issues Associated with Chronic Illness

Any of the issues associated with aging can be seen in those people who are dealing with illness. For example, a person of any age with lung disease may experience difficulty breathing. No matter what the disease or disability, there are two factors which are important to consider when working with people challenged by illness or age. These are **functionality** and **pain.**

Functionality refers to the person's ability to function using the physiologic functions of the body in a normal state or in healthy adaptation to changes. For example, can the person move freely to accomplish daily tasks? If movement is impaired, can she or he get around with the assistance of a cane or walker? Examples of other physiological functions include bladder control, vision, and hearing. Medical care in the form of medications, surgery, nursing care, or other procedures can influence the functionality of the patient, even though disease or age has brought about decline from her or his original level of function.

Pain is the subjective and unpleasant experience derived from sensory stimuli, resulting from immediate damage to the tissues or from long-term functional impairment. It is associated with illness and disease, and has many causes. The sensation of pain may be modified by many factors, including memory, association, and expectation. Treatment of the underlying causes of pain, for example, through surgery or use of drugs, may alleviate pain. However, many people continue to experience chronic pain, which often accompanies loss of function.

There are other physical issues associated with illness and aging that are secondary to the original loss of function:

- **Impaired wound healing.** The aging individual, as well as those suffering from chronic conditions, may experience a slower rate of wound healing.

- **Overuse syndromes.** Loss of physical function of one area may cause overuse of another. For example, a person who uses a wheelchair may have increased pain in the arms and shoulders.
- **Adverse reactions to medications.** Many people experience adverse effects as a result of taking the medications they require to treat the illness. For example, some medications result in dry mouth, nausea, drowsiness, or other unpleasant effects.

Psychosocial Issues Associated with Aging and Illness

Loss of function and physical pain are themselves significant contributors to the psychological issues associated with aging and illness. Loss of physical function in the body leads to other changes for the individual. For example, heart or pulmonary disease may necessitate reduction of physical activities that were once part of an active lifestyle. Debilitating arthritis may force one to give up a pleasant hobby such as knitting or playing the piano. Whereas certain adaptations to changing circumstances may be gradual and easily accepted, others can bring feelings of grief and loss with attendant frustration, sadness, and/or depression.

In addition to the discomfort caused by physical pain, it often contributes to other emotions, such as anxiety and depression. Sometimes the mental and emotional energy consumed in coping with pain leaves the individual fatigued and feeling hopeless. The response to pain can be complex and varied, according to the personality or experience of the individual. For example, the original pain may be the result of tissue damage, but fear of pain leads to increased muscle tension and production of stress hormones, resulting in more pain.

Other psychosocial issues associated with aging and illness include:

- **Loss of mobility.** The individual may find it more difficult to participate in familiar activities. They may lose the ability to drive an automobile and the freedom that comes with it.
- **Changing identity and roles.** Changes in health status are often accompanied by changes in relationships with family, friends, and community. The person may grapple with loss of self-esteem as their self-image and identity undergo change. For example, the person who has enjoyed and taken pride in her or his job or role within a family, finds that she or he can no longer perform the job or play the familiar role. This is a signif-

icant loss for many individuals, which can be either heightened or accommodated, depending on the responses of other people in their lives.

- **Feelings of failure and disappointment.** Individuals may feel disappointed in themselves for failure to "be cured" of their disease. Likewise, they may feel guilt over disappointing others, if they can't seem to recover function. Their sense of self-worth that is attached to achievements and/or goals can suffer as they experience progressive loss of function. Sometimes they display an apologetic attitude to their caregivers based on their level of function or need.
- **Changes of residence.** Often changes in physical functioning necessitate a change of residence. The challenges brought about by aging and illness force the individual to move into a new living situation, which can involve moving into a new home or a new community. It may require adjusting to living with relatives or new caregivers, or becoming part of an assisted living community. While these changes can provide greater safety, better standards of care, and new opportunities for friendship, they also involve letting go of one's past and the feelings of self-determination.
- **Financial concerns.** Generally, as people age, their ability to earn ceases or diminishes, so they are dependent on social security benefits, pensions, or personal savings. The costs of medicine, medical treatments, and personal care become areas of great concern. Circumstances vary widely in the US regarding access to safe and appropriate housing and medical care. Worry and anxiety about paying the bills can greatly affect a person's quality of life.
- **Spiritual issues.** The onset of a major illness, at any age, can challenge a person's core values and beliefs. For example, people who have spent their whole life committed to a healthy lifestyle can be devastated by a diagnosis of a life-threatening illness. "Why me?" they ask. "What did I do wrong? I thought that if I ate well and lived a good life, I could be spared the suffering of this disease." Or they may feel guilty, attributing their illness to mistakes made earlier in their life. They may seek to find blame with other people, government policy, or religious attitudes.
- **Loneliness and isolation.** The loss of function, changing roles, and change of residence can all contribute to feelings of loneliness. People may feel abandoned by friends who once related to them as younger and/or healthy, but now have little time for them. The patient may chose isolation over the fear of rejection by friends or

Hints for Practice

Professional Referrals

It is important for the Comfort Touch practitioner to know when to refer clients to other health care professionals. The medical, psychological, and social issues involved in aging and illness add to the complexity of the physical issues and concerns of the client. Familiarize yourself with the roles of other health care professionals so that you can confer with them and/or refer your clients to them when appropriate. In most medical organizations, including hospices, hospitals, and skilled nursing facilities, patients have access to the expertise of various professionals including: medical specialists, social workers, psychologists, psychiatrists, physical therapists, and chaplains. Remember that as a practitioner of Comfort Touch, you must work only within the limits for which you are adequately trained and/or licensed.

others in their community. Loss of mobility, sight, hearing, and mental cognition all affect the way an individual interacts with others socially (Figure 2-3).

- **Uncertainty**, **unpredictability**, **loss of control.** These are other issues faced by the elderly and the ill. Fear of the unknown and the unpredictable nature of aging, as well as the course of many illnesses, have a depressing effect on many. Some individuals state that loss of control is the biggest challenge they face, frequently a fear greater than death itself. Some have described the uncertainty they feel as "living on borrowed time."

The physical, mental, and emotional facets of the individual can be regarded as inseparable. Care and concern for the person requires respect for the full range of the individual's experience. The practitioner of Comfort Touch is in a position to acknowledge these issues when she or he is a client. For the individual who experiences isolation brought about by loss of function, touch remains an invaluable avenue of connection, easing her or his loneliness, fear, and anxiety.

STORY

Hazel

I am inspired by the resilient spirit I observe in the elderly with whom I work, even as they are challenged by illness, disability, and the changing circumstances of their lives. Hazel was 90 years old when her daughter contacted me. She was hoping that massage could help alleviate the chronic pain her mother experienced as a result of an injury and subsequent surgery to her hip.

Over the next 4 years until the end of her life, I visited Hazel regularly in her home to give her massage. Usually I worked with her lying supine in her bed, making ample use of pillows to help her get comfortable. Sometimes she sat back in her reclining chair, and I pulled up a stool beside her as I worked.

She never remembered my name and often seemed confused about why I had come to her home, but once I began the hands-on session, Hazel responded to my touch as if it were familiar. I felt her sense of trust, as she smiled faintly and closed her watery blue eyes. I noticed the steady quality of her breath as she relaxed, letting go of tension in her body. Her daughter reported that she walked more easily in the days following a massage.

Sometimes, during a session, she drifted in and out of sleep. Other times she recalled stories or sang songs from her childhood. When touching her I could feel a

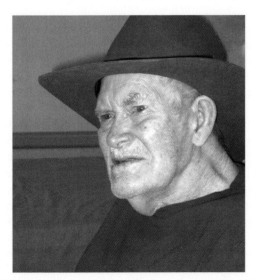

FIGURE 2-3. Resident of a skilled nursing facility. This elderly man, once physically strong and active, displays a look of bewilderment at the changes in his life.

quality in her body's tissues that spoke to me of her many years of hard work on the family farm. Even as I comforted her with soothing touch, I could appreciate the love and care she had provided for so many others in her long and full life.

She seldom commented on the therapy itself, but one day as I held her hand to massage it, she said, "That sure does feel good. Why, I believe I could play the piano."

I looked at her a little surprised and replied, "Hazel, I didn't know you played the piano."

She laughed. "Oh, I never could before!"

 ## Bereavement—Dealing with Grief and Loss

Bereavement is the process of reacting to loss. The word *bereave* derives from root words meaning "to break or rend apart; to rob." The bereaved individual feels robbed or deprived of someone or something familiar and valuable. **Grief** is the suffering or distress experienced because of a loss. Derived from Latin words meaning "to burden" or "heavy," grief involves a complex set of emotions, including sadness, fear, regret, and yearning for what was lost. The person experiencing grief is affected physically, emotionally, and mentally (Figure 2-4).

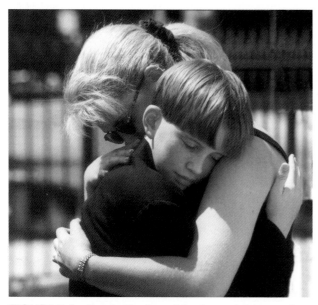

FIGURE 2-4. Comforting hug. A brother and sister comfort each other as they mourn the death of their father.

Understanding Grief as a Response to Loss

Bereavement is most often thought of as the mourning associated with losses caused by death, but the process of grieving can be applied to many other life-changing events, including disability, divorce, job loss, financial loss, or other changes in physical circumstances or relationships. Aging itself is a process involving many changes, including losses for which a person may grieve. A person living with chronic illness or disability may undergo an extensive process of grieving over the loss of health or function.

Whether a loss is sudden and specific, as with a death, or prolonged, as with a gradual loss of function owing to illness, it is normal for the individual to move through a range of responses and reactions. While Sigmund Freud pioneered the study of bereavement in his essay "Mourning and Melancholia," written in 1917, it was psychiatrist Elizabeth Kubler-Ross who advanced the study of bereavement in relation to the dying process. In her groundbreaking book "On Death and Dying," published in 1969, she proposed five psychological stages of dying: denial, anger, bargaining, depression, and, finally, acceptance. Her passionate commitment to ease the psychological as well as physical suffering of the ill and dying compelled her to work to bring about awareness of these issues within the mainstream of medicine and psychology. Her work paralleled the growing hospice movement, which sought to bring compassion and dignity to the terminally ill.

British psychiatrist John Bowlby's study of attachment behavior in children contributed to the understanding of bereavement. His theory of attachment, presented in the 1960s, provided an explanation for the common human tendency to develop strong affectional bonds. Grief is an instinctive universal response to separation.[2] Together with psychiatrist Colin Parkes in their study of adult grieving, they described four phases of grief, which involved the experiences of numbness with intermittent anger; yearning; disorganization and despair; and organization.[3]

Understanding of the grieving process has continued to expand as it applies not only to death and dying, but also to the broader range of human experience. Grieving is *not* a simple linear process. It applies not only to losses incurred as a result of death or the anticipation of death, but also to other kinds of losses. For example, grief can be experienced when someone is diagnosed with a life-threatening and/or debilitating disease. The physical and psychosocial issues involved with aging and illness also contribute to the complexity of the bereavement process for many individuals.

More recent advances in the understanding of grief theory include the dual process model developed by

Margaret Stroebe and Henk Schut.[4] While previous models focus on stages and phases of grieving, the dual-process model recognizes a dynamic in which the bereaved individual alternates between focusing on the loss—with all of the associated reactions and responses—and avoiding focusing on the loss in order to cope with the stresses and requirements of everyday life. In this model it is recognized that both expressing and controlling emotion have value for the individual who is dealing with loss. The bereaved person is able to take time off from the intensity of emotional response to the loss in order to deal with the life changes brought about by the loss.

The Cycle of Grief

How individuals respond to loss depends on many factors, including their personal belief systems, social and cultural conditioning, practical coping skills, and their existing familial and social support networks. While people experience grief in many possible ways, there are general patterns of emotions and reactions that occur at various stages after the loss. The Cycle of Grief pictured here is a useful image for individuals to understand their own responses to loss. For the practitioners of Comfort Touch it is also a helpful way to understand the psychosocial experiences of their clients, as they move from the initial reactions to loss through a myriad of possible reactions and emotions, toward a healthy adaptation to change (Figure 2-5).

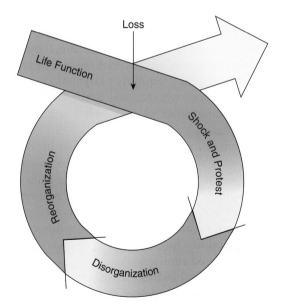

FIGURE 2-5. The cycle of grief. This image provides a helpful way to understand the experiences of grieving individuals as they move through a myriad of possible reactions and responses to the loss, toward adaptation to change.

Consistent with the understanding of the dual-process model of grieving, keep in mind that even as people exhibit the range of reactions and responses shown in the cycle of grief, they may also "take time off" from feeling in order to respond to their practical needs in everyday life. For example, someone who has lost a loved one might still need to care for young children in the family, so will set aside her or his own feelings in order to attend to the needs of others. They may also take a break from the intensity of emotion through other self-care measures that can include nutrition, rest, exercise, massage, and/or social interaction.

Shock, Protest

The first stage following a loss is characterized by *shock* and *protest.* In the initial hours, days, or weeks following a loss, the individual may experience *numbness* or actively protest the reality of the loss. *Denial* is a way that many people protect themselves from the painful reality of their new situation. They may feel *anxiety* and *fear*, with attendant feelings of uncertainty or confusion. *Sadness, loneliness*, and intense *yearning* for whom or what was lost are common experiences.

The bereaved individual may also experience *relief* if, for example, the death of a loved one occurred after a long and painful illness. *Joy* may be felt where death is believed to be a release into a freer or happier state of being. Other kinds of loss can bring a feeling a relief, because the uncertainty of waiting has ended.

Another common reaction is *anger*, which may be a feeling of frustration directed toward oneself or others. *Guilt* may be present for some, as often occurs when death is by accident or suicide, and the survivors wonder what they could have done to prevent it. *Regret* is another feeling that occurs when the individual wishes she or he had made different choices earlier in her or his life. For example, someone who has suffered from a debilitating accident or been diagnosed with a major illness may wish they had made different lifestyle choices.

The bereaved may try to "*bargain*" their way out of the loss. In other words, they may promise to change their ways to regain what was lost, whether that loss was a change in their own health status, a change in a relationship, or the loss through death of a loved one.

Some individuals *idealize* whom or what they have lost, refusing to acknowledge the full reality of the person or their prior situation. Conversely, some people *demonize* whom or what they have lost, as is sometimes the case with people as they go through the process of separation or divorce.

Physical reactions and symptoms may include *insomnia, crying, muscle weakness, nausea*, and/or *loss of appetite.* Some people experience *difficulty breathing.*

Grief itself can be experienced as *physical pain* and has been described in many ways, including the following words applied to various parts of the body: dull, aching, stinging, biting, sharp, pressure, contracted, or constricted. Any or all of these reactions are considered a normal part of grieving. Just as people are distinct in how they respond to everyday stresses and challenges of life, so will they respond in different ways to loss. Some feelings or reactions may be fleeting; others will be of persistent intensity.

The Comfort Touch practitioner best serves grieving individuals by allowing them to be present with their feelings. It is not necessary to diagnose bereaved people or judge their process; rather is it most respectful to simply be present and listen, acknowledging the significance of their experiences. If the client seems to be exhibiting reactions or behaviors outside of a normal range, it is wise to refer her or him for further evaluation and/or counseling with a mental health professional.

Disorganization

The next stage in the cycle of grief is characterized by *disorganization*. The loss has occurred and the initial shock has begun to wear off, but now the individual is left to cope with a reality that is different. Life is not organized the way it was before. The sense of disorganization occurs on different levels.

Disorganization often involves practical concerns, which may include financial and legal issues. Mentally, the individual can feel disoriented and overwhelmed with decisions to make. Sometimes even the simplest decision seems to take an inordinate amount of energy. They may experience *forgetfulness,* or in some cases, become obsessive in their behavior, thinking, or feeling.

Emotionally, some feelings may persist or intensify from the first phase. Some feelings may shift and change, giving way to others. The range of emotions that might be felt during this time includes *anger, sadness, depression, despair, anguish,* and *low self-esteem. Physical exhaustion* tends to intensify many of these feelings.

Socially, the person who is grieving may feel *detached, withdrawn, apathetic,* or *anti-social.* Some may feel very needy and afraid to be alone. Disorganization also occurs within the family or social network of the bereaved individual. Differences in the way people communicate and deal with loss within the social group may vary, contributing added pressures and distress to the individual.

Periods of grief are difficult times for people. In its intensity, grieving may last for several weeks or months, sometimes years. Whereas people often have the support of family and friends soon after a loss, they are often alone in their grief as time goes on. Typically, our culture does not give people time to grieve. Furthermore, it is not customary to talk about our most significant losses or share our feelings with the people we work with or interact with socially. Without adequate support during this time, bereaved people feel further alienation and the added burden of suffering their grief alone. In this time, Comfort Touch can provide much needed support, providing a steady and nurturing presence.

Reorganization

With time, the acute pain of loss begins to subside, and the bereaved individual begins to *reorganize* their life. Painful emotions do carry over into this phase, but the intensity or duration of the feeling is usually less than in the previous phases. One begins to accept or understand that the loss is permanent, and begins to adapt to a new life, integrating the reality of the changes into their present life.

The process of reorganization involves changes and adaptations on many levels. When the loss involves the death of a loved one, the survivor learns to reorganize his or her life physically, emotionally, and mentally without the presence of that special person. When the loss involves illness or disability, the person learns to adjust their physical surroundings, lifestyle, and health care to the current situation.

Loss of one kind—either of person, place, or quality of life—involves changes in other activities and relationships. For example, the person who is injured in a debilitating accident may find it difficult or impossible to participate in once-enjoyable activities such as hiking or skiing. As they reorganize their life, they might find other activities they enjoy that are less physically demanding. Or if they regularly participated in activities with a loved one who has now left or died, they can adapt by finding other people with whom to enjoy social activities.

Reorganization and adaptation also involve an appreciation of the pleasant and/or valued memories of the past, while accepting the reality of the present circumstance. It becomes easier to celebrate and remember the past without feeling intense sadness. Many people learn the value of compassion, while opening to new possibilities for social connection with others who have suffered similar losses.

As the bereaved individual adapts to the change, they may begin to feel improved self-esteem and mental clarity. It becomes easier to make decisions and engage with others socially. Physical exhaustion gives way to renewed energy and confidence.

Variables in the Expression of Grief

While the grief cycle is portrayed here as one phase that occurs after another, it is *not* a fixed process, either in length of time, intensity, or sequence of emotional expression. The cycle shows the range of experience of people going through the normal process of grieving. Not only do people vary in their responses to loss, but they may react differently to different losses. Multiple losses complicate the picture. A person may be in one phase with one loss and in another phase with another loss. Or the experience of one loss may trigger unresolved feelings of a prior loss. The individual may think they have come through the cycle only to experience an upsurge of anguished feelings, sometimes around an anniversary, birthday, or holiday.

Adaptation to Change

As the individual moves through the process of grieving, he or she may realize that loss is neither good nor bad, right nor wrong. Change and loss are inevitable aspects of human experience. The pain of loss may never fully go away, but the individual learns to adapt to change. Helen Keller said, "What we have once enjoyed we can never lose. All we love deeply becomes a part of us." Her words illustrate the concept of healthy adaptation to change and loss. It is our role as practitioners of Comfort Touch to provide a safe, open-hearted, non-judgmental, and reassuring atmosphere to the bereaved individual.

Summary

- While health generally refers to a state of wholeness, free of physical, mental, or emotional infirmity, the concept of health also refers to the ability of the individual to adapt to the changes brought about by age, life circumstance, illness, or injury.
- The intention to cure implies a need to fix or change the circumstance of the patient. The intention to heal emphasizes the acknowledgment of the individual as a whole human being, regardless of her or his current condition or diagnosis.
- The National Center for Complementary and Alternative Medicine (NCCAM) defines three categories of medicine: conventional medicine, alternative medicine, and complementary medicine.
- Comfort Touch is a valuable complement to conventional medicine as well as a therapeutic model of massage, grounded in a tradition of nurturing touch.

- Physical issues of aging and/or illness involve changes and/or loss of function to the various tissues, organs, and systems of the body. Pain is a serious issue for many affected by age, illness, and injury.
- Losses of function and/or physical pain are significant contributors to the psychosocial issues associated with aging and illness. Other issues include depression, anxiety, financial concerns, isolation, and loneliness.
- Bereavement is the process of dealing with losses associated with change including: death, divorce, financial loss, or changes in physical circumstances and relationships.
- The Cycle of Grief describes the range of emotions and responses a person may have in reaction to loss. The primary phases are characterized by shock and protest, disorganization, and reorganization.
- People vary in their expressions of grief and their ability to adapt to changes brought about by aging, illness, and other losses in life. Comfort Touch offers a respectful and nurturing therapy to assist others to experience a sense of well-being in the midst of life challenges.

Review Questions

1. What qualities characterize physical, mental, or emotional health? How do you define health?
2. What is the difference between acute illness and chronic illness? Give examples of each.
3. What is the difference between healing and curing?
4. Describe the three categories of medicine defined by the National Center for Complementary and Alternative Medicine (NCCAM). Give an example of each.
5. How is Comfort Touch used as a complement to conventional medicine?
6. List five or more physical changes that occur with aging. For example, what are the effects of aging on the skin, the cardiovascular system, the respiratory system, etc.?
7. Give examples of changes in functionality experienced by those with chronic illness.
8. List five or more psychosocial issues associated with aging and illness.
9. List five examples of loss for which a person might grieve. What have been the most significant losses in your own life?
10. What are the three primary phases of the Cycle of Grief?

References

1. The US Administration on Aging. *A Profile of Older Americans: 2006*. Washington, DC: Department of Health and Human Services. http://www.aoa.gov/prof/Statistics/profile/2006/4.asp?pf=true. Accessed June, 2007.
2. Dent A. Supporting the bereaved: theory and practice. *Counseling at Work*. 2005;Autumn:22–23.
3. Bretherton I. The origins of attachment theory: John Bowlby and Mary Ainsworth. *Dev Psychol*. 1992;28:759–775.
4. Stroebe M, Schut H. The dual process model of coping with bereavement: rationale and description. *Death Stud*. 1999;23(3):197–224.

Suggested Reading

Alami GB. Relationship of CAM and conventional medicine: past, present, future [monograph online]. Montreal, QB: McGill University; July 2000. http://sprojects.mmi. mcgill. ca/cam/relationship.htm. Accessed January 3, 2005.

Beers MH, Merkow R, eds. *The Merck Manual of Geriatrics*. 3rd ed. Whitehouse Station, NJ: Merck & Company; 2000.

Bowlby J. *Attachment and Loss: Loss, Sadness, and Depression*. Vol. 3. New York: Basic Books; 1980.

Brooke E. *Medicine Women: A Pictorial History of Women Healers*. Wheaton, IL: Quest Books; 1997.

Duff K. *The Alchemy of Illness*. New York: Bell Tower; 1993.

Frank A. *At the Will of the Body—Reflections on Illness*. Boston, MA: Houghton Mifflin; 1991.

Freud S. *Mourning and Melancholia. The Complete Psychological Works of Sigmund Freud:* Vol. 8. London: Vintage; 2001.

Holmes J. *John Bowlby and Attachment Theory*. London: Routledge; 1993.

Hufford D. Cultural and social perspectives on alternative medicine: background and assumptions. *Alternative Therapies*. 1995;1(1):53–61.

Kubler-Ross E. *On Death and Dying*. New York: Touchstone; 1969.

Nelson D. *Making Friends with Cancer*. Findhorn, Scotland: Findhorn Press; 2000.

Parkes CM. *Bereavement: Studies of Grief in Adult Life*. New York: International University Press; 1972.

Rando T. *How To Go On Living When Someone You Love Dies*. Lanham, MD: Lexington Books; 1988.

Weed S. *Healing Wise—Wise Woman Herbal*. Woodstock, NY: Ash Tree Publishing; 1989.

Weed S. *New Menopausal Years: The Wise Woman Way*. Woodstock, NY: Ash Tree Publishing; 2002.

Worden W. *Grief Counseling and Grief Therapy; A Handbook for the Mental Health Practitioner*. New York: Springer Publishing Company, Inc.; 1991.

Approaching the Client

> For an hour I felt like I was the most important person in the world.
> —Brenda Swede, Comfort Touch client

A Comfort Touch session provides the client with the opportunity to receive special attention that can enhance the quality of her or his health and well-being. The practitioner of this therapy needs to have an understanding of the physical and emotional needs of the client, along with skill in appropriate hands-on technique. This chapter will focus on factors that contribute to an enjoyable and rewarding experience for both the client and practitioner. These include adherence to specific protocols for hygiene, communication with the client, and creation of a safe and healing atmosphere. Documentation of the session will also be discussed.

The practitioner of Comfort Touch instills confidence in the client by adherence to professional standards of conduct, as well as attention to details that make clients feel safe, comfortable, and acknowledged for their value as human beings. The offering of touch to the elderly or the ill is based on the desire of the health care provider to communicate caring and compassion for the person receiving it. Figure 3-1 shows how a comforting touch at the beginning of social worker's visit can be used to convey concern for the client and place him at ease.

Roles and Responsibilities for Comfort Touch Practitioners

The roles and responsibilities of practitioners of Comfort Touch will vary somewhat, depending on the setting in

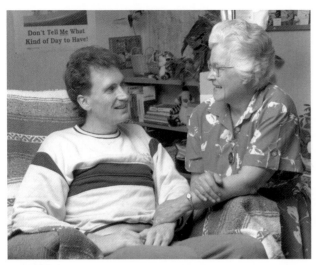

FIGURE 3-1. **Caring Touch.** A hospice social worker establishes rapport with her patient, placing him at ease as she gently touches his arm.

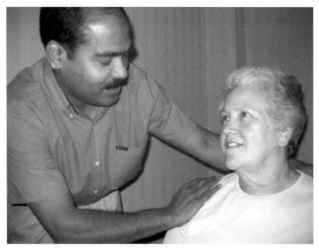

FIGURE 3-2. **Scope of practice.** This physical therapist uses techniques of Comfort Touch to help a patient relax before beginning therapeutic exercises on her shoulder.

which they work and the professional **scope of practice** to which they are bound. The following are general guidelines to follow.

- **Trainings.** Complete all training and orientation required for the setting in which you work, whether as a regular member of the staff or as a part-time or contract employee. Training requirements for certification and/or licensing for massage therapists vary from state to state, so check to make sure you are in compliance with local regulations. Also complete the necessary training in Comfort Touch technique before beginning to practice it.

- **Scope of Practice.** Observe the scope of practice of your profession. For example, if you are a massage therapist, you may *not* diagnose medical conditions or prescribe medical treatments. Be aware that different medical settings and/or organizations will specify which practices suit your training. For example, in a hospital setting, a massage therapist usually requires the assistance of nursing staff to reposition a patient, particularly if lifting of the patient is involved. Professions such as nursing or physical therapy do involve touching a patient, so Comfort Touch can easily be incorporated into their scope of practice. Figure 3-2 shows a physical therapist who uses Comfort Touch to help a client relax before beginning a session of therapeutic exercises.

- **Hygiene and Universal Precautions.** Understand and observe all rules of hygiene. Wash your hands and forearms thoroughly, using soap and running water, before and after touching the patient. Make sure that your fingernails are clean and short. Avoid wearing rings, bracelets, or watches during the hands-on session. Understand and observe rules of **Standard** and **Universal Precautions.** These are precautions set forth by the Centers for Disease Control and Prevention which are designed to reduce the risk of transmission of microorganisms from both recognized and unrecognized sources of infection in hospitals and other medical settings. They involve the use of protective barriers such as gloves, gowns, masks, or protective eyewear to reduce the risk of exposure of the health care worker's skin or mucous membranes to potentially infectious materials. See Appendix A.

- **Tuberculosis testing and infectious diseases.** Health care workers are required to show proof of tuberculosis testing. Do not work if you know you have an infectious illness; for example, a cold or influenza. Some facilities require proof of other immunizations.

- **Professionalism.** Wear clean and appropriate attire. Refrain from using alcohol or drugs. Act in a respectful manner at all times.

- **Timeliness.** Be on time for all appointments or scheduled times of work. Be prompt in returning phone calls when arranging schedules with staff or clients.

- **Confidentiality.** To protect the privacy of your clients, observe strict rules of confidentiality. Conversations about the client as well as written records are to be shared only with authorized people who are directly involved in the patient's care. Written notes need to be kept in a safe place where they are protected from anyone else's view. Breaching of confidentiality is an unethical behavior and a serious violation of a person's privacy.

- **Insurance.** You may be required to carry personal professional liability insurance. Provide documentation, if necessary.
- **Documentation.** Complete all required documentation of the session for the setting in which you work. (See Chapter 7, Communication and Documentation in the Healthcare System.)
- **Self-Care.** It is the responsibility of the practitioner to be mindful of her or his own self-care in terms of matters of health and wellness. For example, pay attention to your own needs relative to good nutrition, exercise and rest, and management of stress. Your attitude about self-care imparts a sense of confidence to the client.
- **Personal mental preparation and grounding.** It is helpful to take a few moments before beginning a session to mentally prepare to be with the client. The concept of *grounding* is helpful, as you envision yourself connected to the earth beneath you. Grounding is a state of being in which the individual is confident in her or his skills, and carries a sense of stability and connection to the earth. When you are well-grounded, you have a greater ability to tune into the world around you, and still maintain a focus to work and communicate clearly with others. Grounding helps you to establish and maintain rapport with your clients. If you are personally grounded, you inspire a sense of confidence and groundedness in others. (See Chapter 8 for specific self-care and grounding exercises.)

Before the Session

Before beginning the hands-on session, it is important to have authorization to touch the client. If the client is in a medical setting, you will usually need to check in with the supervising nurse or other administrator before the session. Also, you must have adequate information regarding the patient's physical health and state of mind, if you are to work safely and appropriately. The following are guidelines for approaching the client, and include intake and assessment, communication skills, precautions in the use of touch, and factors that contribute to a healing environment.

Medical Intake and Client Information

If you are working in a medical setting (ie, hospice, hospital, skilled nursing facility, or rehabilitation center), you may have direct access to the medical records of a patient. If so, consult the patient's chart to see her or his age, medical diagnosis, and other relevant information.

If you are working with a private client, you will take your own client information. Client intake includes relevant personal contact information, medical history, and a listing of current health concerns. It contains a listing of medications being taken, and other therapies being utilized by the patient, such as physical therapy or occupational therapy. It also contains the stated reason for receiving the massage. Refer to Figure 7-1 for a sample of a Client Information form.

The Client Information form may be filled out in one of the following three ways:

1. **The client fills out the form.** In a general massage practice, the client may fill out the form before a massage session. If so, the therapist should look it over and verify the information with the individual. Notice what is relevant to the session, and ask additional questions to clarify or elaborate on any of the information.
2. **The massage therapist completes the form during an interview with the client.** As the client responds to the questions, the massage therapist records these answers, gathering the information necessary to offer a safe and appropriate session. By asking the questions in a clear and direct manner, the therapist helps to build rapport with the client.
3. **A health care provider or patient caregiver completes the form.** If the client is a hospital or hospice patient, much of the information will have been recorded in the patient's chart by their health care providers. The massage therapist can add relevant information to the chart, as necessary. Follow-up by asking the patient to verify the information. In some instances, the patient will not be able to speak or communicate clearly, so it is up to the therapist to get all relevant information from the health care provider (eg, a nurse) or family member. This would be the case, for example, with the patient who has dementia or another debilitating condition, such as stroke or Parkinson's disease that affects the ability to communicate.

You can use the form provided in Chapter 7 (Figure 7-1) to record patient information, or use it as a guide and adapt it to the setting and situation in which you are working. There are three primary components to gathering information before beginning hands-on work:

1. **Contact information.** This includes the client's name, address, phone number, and date of birth. If the individual is in a medical setting other than her or his own home, record both home address and the room number for the facility where the person is currently staying.

You may also need to record the name and address of a responsible family member, if you are also communicating with her or him.

2. **Medical history.** This includes a listing and summary of illnesses, injuries, surgeries, and other medical conditions or concerns. A medical history includes both past and current conditions, as well as medical requirements for treatments and medications. For example, it may include "Chronic Obstructive Pulmonary Disease (COPD), requiring regular use of oxygen." It also includes notations about the client's level of activity and mobility; for example, "The client has limited mobility, requiring the use of a wheelchair; needs assistance for positioning in bed." Note the client's ability to communicate and the condition of the special senses of sight and hearing. A medical history also lists current medications and other treatments being used, such as physical therapy.

3. **Needs for massage therapy.** Whether the patient is self-referred or referred by another health care professional or family member, the client information form will record the reasons for requesting massage therapy or Comfort Touch. These reasons include, but are not limited to the following: general relaxation; pain relief; general or specific muscular tension; relief from loneliness, depression, or anxiety; and/or general health maintenance.

Introduction and Communication

Your initial introduction to the client sets the tone for the session to come. It will precede the taking of the client information if you are interviewing the client directly. In working with the elderly and the ill, special sensitivity is required in communication. Be mindful that many people may be affected by visual or auditory impairment. It is helpful to enter the room slowly, allowing them time to adjust to your presence. Walk up to the individual and introduce yourself. For example: "Hello, my name is Sarah. I am the massage therapist here with hospice." Give the patient a moment to take in that information. "I am here to give you a Comfort Touch session. Is that okay with you now?" With these few words you (1) introduce yourself, (2) state your intention in offering touch, and (3) ask for the patient's consent to be touched. The massage therapist shown in Figure 3-3 greets her client who lives in a skilled nursing facility.

Here are some tips on communication with the elderly and/or the ill:

- **Speak slowly and clearly, looking directly at the person.** Speaking slowly gives the individ-

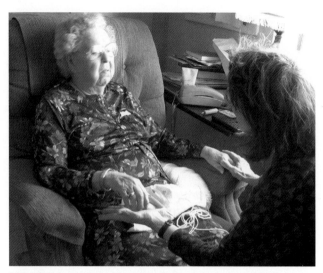

FIGURE 3-3. Greeting the client. The massage therapist greets Helen, aged 99, a regular client accustomed to receiving Comfort Touch while sitting in her recliner in a skilled nursing facility. The therapist establishes eye contact as she asks Helen what she needs from the session. The client has set aside her crocheting project while voicing her interest in receiving some pain relief for her hands.

ual time to adjust to your presence, as well as to process the words you are speaking.

- **Speak loudly enough.** Remember that many elderly people have some degree of hearing loss.

- **Use individuals' names when addressing them.** The common practice is to use their first names, but you may ask how they prefer to be addressed. For example, Anne Smith, may prefer to be addressed as "Mrs. Smith," "Anne," or "Annie." Avoid terms of endearment, such as "dear." Respectfully using a person's name of choice gets her attention, and assures the greatest level of response from her in the moment.

- **Do not make assumptions about what they do or do not understand.** Just because someone does not answer you directly does not mean that she or he do not understand what you are saying.

- Introduce yourself even if the person appears to be asleep or incoherent. You will be surprised at how often she or he respond, and are glad that you have come.

- **Give the person time to respond, before continuing to speak.** Remember that the person affected by age, disease processes, or medication may need more time to mentally process what you have said, and to formulate a verbal or nonverbal response.

- **Choose language appropriately.** Be mindful to use language that is familiar to the client. Avoid using slang, jargon, or overcomplicated explanations of what you are doing. Many older people will reject an offer of "massage," but will be open to an offer of "comfort touch," or a "foot rub." There are still many who associate negative connotations with the word "massage."

Precautions in the Use of Touch

With proper training and supervision, Comfort Touch techniques can be used even with the most fragile or seriously ill patient. Using the principles described herein, the practitioner will find a way to touch the individual who is open to receiving the benefits of touch. The contact can be very simple. For example, it might involve holding the hand, or gently holding and encompassing the feet.

There are some conditions, however, where touch is *not* recommended for specific areas or parts of the body. Avoid touching:

- The site of tumors or lumps
- The site of a recent surgery
- **Deep vein thrombosis** (This is a blood clot that develops in a deep vein, usually in the leg. Because of the potential of DVTs to develop after surgery, it is advised to avoid massage below the waist, unless cleared by a physician.)
- Phlebitis (inflammation of a vein)
- Fractures
- Burns, rashes, undiagnosed or contagious skin problems, or areas of skin irritation
- Open sore or injuries
- Areas of infection or inflammation
- *Any* area that is painful to the touch
- Areas of acute pain, or pain of unknown origin

Use caution in working with people with the following conditions. In these situations, it is best to have further training and/or the guidance of a qualified health professional, who can assess the situation. The client is often able to tell you if touch is helpful. For example, for a client with arthritic hands, it may be helpful for the therapist to hold the hands, letting the warmth of contact bring relief, while avoiding pressure which could contribute to more pain.

- Arthritis
- Headaches
- Dizziness
- Nausea
- Fever
- Edema

The following are a few other important considerations requiring awareness and caution:

- **Be especially careful with massage of the neck.** Use particular caution when working on the neck, using only broad contact. Do *not* use specific pressure into the neck itself. The bony structures of the neck—the spinous and transverse processes—and the blood vessels are too vulnerable to warrant working into them without specific training. Most often, patients who report pain in the neck will find relief of that pain if the therapist uses Comfort Touch techniques (*broad encompassing contact pressure* and *contact circling*) on the trapezius muscles, with particular attention to the belly of the trapezius. Also, *contact pressure* and *contact circling* along the occipital ridge are safe and effective ways to alleviate neck pain.
- **Avoid the prone (face down) position.** Most often, massage of the elderly and the ill is performed in the supine (face up), side-lying, or seated positions. The prone position is difficult because of a client's a) lack of flexibility in the neck, b) impaired breathing, c) impaired circulation in the neck, and d) greater difficulty to communicate feedback to the therapist. (Even in healthy individuals, the use of the prone position on a massage table contributes to respiratory congestion and impaired breathing. The use of a face cradle often makes this condition worse.)
- **Respect a patient's wishes regarding touch.** If the client does not want to be touched in a particular place, respect that request. If the person's condition has markedly changed since your last visit, talk to the health care provider (physician, nurse, or nurse's aide) or family caregiver before proceeding with the massage. Sometimes the client will not want to be touched at all. At other times, the client will be grateful to be touched, if only to have a hand held, or to receive a simple foot massage.
- **Use caution in the use of scents.** Be aware of reasons to avoid the use of scents in both massage lotions and in aerial sprays. Many body care products contain chemicals that can cause irritation and/or allergic reactions. These may be synthetic chemicals or natural essential oils. Strong scents that are enjoyed by one person may be unpleasant to another, so avoid making assumptions. Remember that the techniques of Comfort Touch do not require the use of lotion or oil on the skin. For more information on this subject see Appendix B.

Creating a Safe and Healing Environment

Before beginning the hands-on part of a Comfort Touch massage session, it is important to assess the setting. Whether the session takes place in a medical or a home-care setting, there are a number of factors to consider that will contribute to the experience of safety and the atmosphere of healing for the patient.

The Physical Setting

When entering the client's room, be attentive to factors involving the safety or comfort of the client:

- **Electrical and/or medical equipment.** Look around the room. Are there electrical cords in sight for lamps or medical equipment? Is there tubing for oxygen tanks, or tubing for other medical devices such as intravenous drips, catheters, or emergency buttons? Are there pads on the floor for safety? (In some skilled nursing facilities, the hospital beds are lowered to within a foot of floor level and foam pads are used beside the bed, in order to avoid the use of safety rails.)
- **The bed or chair for the client.** Comfort Touch is often given to the patient who is in her or his own bed, which may be a regular bed or a hospital bed. The client may also be in a recliner or a comfortable chair.
- **Massage tables.** For the safety and comfort of the client, it is generally advised *not* to use a massage table. Getting on a table can be difficult, even dangerous, to the medically fragile client, and the typical massage table is much too narrow and hard to be comfortable. Sometimes it is feasible for a client in initial sessions to get onto a massage table, only to find it increasingly difficult to negotiate as their illness or disability progresses. So it is best to avoid this potential association of massage with a table, as it creates another sense of loss for the individual as they lose mobility.
- **Other furniture.** The comfort of patients is paramount. As the therapist, you will learn how to adjust to their situation *without* compromising your own comfort. You might need to move small tables or other furniture to allow easier access to the client. It is advisable to use a small stool to allow you to sit close to the patient's bed or chair. A stool like the one pictured in Figure 3-4 is lightweight, stable, and easy to move around. It can fit in close quarters in a patient's home or in the medical setting. A footstool can also be utilized; it is helpful when sitting at the foot of the bed to massage the client's feet.

The Atmosphere and Intention of Healing

Before beginning the hands-on part of a session, be attentive to factors that contribute to a healing atmosphere. Respect the wishes of clients about their preferences. Here are some things to consider:

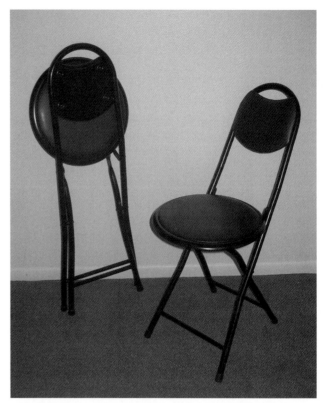

FIGURE 3-4. Lightweight, folding metal stool. An inexpensive but valuable tool, a small folding metal stool can be a great help to the Comfort Touch practitioner who works in homecare and medical settings. It can be purchased at hardware stores and home centers.

- **The temperature of the room.** Make thermostatic adjustments according to the patient's need. Add blankets to the bed if needed for warmth.
- **Air flow.** Notice if there is a comfortable degree of circulating air. Open or close windows and doors or adjust fans, as needed.
- **Lighting.** Indirect lighting is preferable to overhead lighting as it is more conducive to relaxation. Illumination should be adequate to ensure the physical and psychological safety of both the client and the therapist. Windows can provide pleasant, natural lighting, as well as a view to the outside world. Be aware, however, that patients with certain medical conditions may be extremely sensitive to light.
- **Music.** Some clients enjoy having music played during their Comfort Touch session. They may have their own audio equipment and CDs or audiocassettes, or you may provide them. Some clients who are used to playing the radio or television may wish to leave it on, or they may prefer to turn it off. Let this choice be the

prerogative of the client. For some the familiarity of sounds is comforting; for others, it is a distraction. Those with hearing impairment might even find the sound of music to be annoying.

- **Scent.** Notice the smells in the room. Does it smell clean? Your sense of smell can alert you to hygiene issues that need to be addressed. If you are working in a medical facility, you may need to check with staff to see that the patient's personal hygienic needs are addressed before beginning the massage.

  Use scents, in lotion or in the air, only with extreme caution, in order to avoid irritation to the client's skin, mucous membranes, eyes, or respiratory passages and lungs. Sometimes a simple scent, such as a few fresh flowers (eg, rose, carnation, stock, lavender) can add to the beauty and enjoyment of the setting. Notice the client's response to anything new that you introduce to the setting.

- **Candles.** Avoid the use of candles. They present an unnecessary safety hazard around medical equipment and normal household or bedside items. Many candles produce toxic fumes when burned.

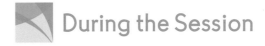

During the Session

During a Comfort Touch session, there are a number of factors that complement the quality of the hands-on work. These include concerns about the appropriate positioning of the patient, body patterning for the therapist, ongoing communication, and other pertinent details regarding draping, use of lotions, and the length of the session. Remember that the Comfort Touch approach is *client-centered*, whereby the needs of the client are acknowledged and, whenever possible, should influence treatment and communication choices made by the therapist. For example, the client chooses the position for the massage session, and the therapist adapts to that choice. Likewise, conversation is focused primarily on the needs and interests of the client, not those of the therapist.

Positioning the Client

Comfort Touch can be offered to the client who is lying in a standard bed, or a hospital bed. The client might also be in a chair, wheelchair, or recliner. Each of these options presents particular advantages and

Hints for Practice

Establishing Rapport

In a typical massage practice the client comes into the therapist's office, who gets to know the person by asking questions of her or him in an intake interview. When working with the elderly and/or the chronically ill, there can be limitations to the client's ability to communicate, so the practitioner of Comfort Touch is often challenged to establish rapport in other ways.

One way to get to know clients is by observing their surroundings, whether they are in a private home or a room in a residential care facility, a hospice, or other medical setting. Notice photographs or greeting cards that are in the room that can tell you something about the person and her or his life. Your comment about a photo that you see can evoke a fond memory for the client about a special loved one, or a particularly happy time.

As you observe the photos, artworks or special objects in a client's room, you develop a greater appreciation for the wholeness of the person's life. Your words of interest or appreciation about what you see lets her or him know that you see the person beyond the frail individual she or he now appears to be. For example, when I commented to one elderly woman about a photo of a sailboat on her wall, she began to tell me about her deceased husband, and all the happy times they and their children had shared in that boat.

In one skilled nursing facility, I worked with an elderly man with Parkinson's disease. He had limited ability to speak, and seemed distant and uncommunicative. I noticed that he had a single framed photograph on the wall. It was of a young man hiking on a trail in steep mountainous terrain. When I asked if that was him in the photo, he smiled and nodded his head, indicating that it was. The photo helped me to see him as a whole person, one who carried that memory and experience of the wilderness into the present. As I shared my love of the mountains with him, he listened attentively, grateful to be seen and acknowledged.

challenges. The therapist must always be attentive to the safety and comfort of patients, and be flexible in adapting to their needs in order to provide the most effective work. Be sensitive to the varying degrees of mobility of the clients and allow them to move any part of their body to be most comfortable. Your attitude is important—you want them to feel encouraged about what they can do, not discouraged about their limitations.

The following are considerations for positioning the client for a massage session.

Hospital Bed—Supine Position

The hospital bed offers a number of advantages for both the client and the therapist. It allows for a number of adjustments that can be made for the client's comfort, as well as offering easy access for the practitioner. Hospital beds vary in the way they function, so it is always advisable to have a caregiver of the client or other staff member assist you in working with the bed. Most often the client will be in the supine position, that is, *face up* in the bed. Adjustments can be made to elevate the head and upper body of the patient, as well as to elevate the legs. The bed may also have height adjustments. Side rails can be lowered during a session. Foot boards can often be removed to allow for easier access to massage the feet. Figure 3-5 shows a patient receiving Comfort Touch in a hospital bed.

Standard Bed—Supine Position

A standard bed can be adapted for the patient's comfort, as shown in Figure 3-6. For the client who benefits by having the head and upper body elevated (ie, someone with impaired breathing), two or three pillows can be used as props on the bed. When elevating the upper body, make sure that the head remains in correct alignment with the back. A small towel, such as the one shown in Figure 3-7 can be used to support the neck.

Pillows that are placed under the knees allow greater comfort for the client's back, prevent hyperextension of the knees, and contribute to relaxation of the legs. Small towels may be rolled and used under the client's ankles to make sure that the heel bones are not rubbing on the bed and causing pressure sores. Additionally, small towels or pillows can be used under the arms to provide support or comfort.

Hospital or Standard Bed—Side-Lying Position

The side-lying position is sometimes preferred, as it allows easy access to the back, and can be an especially comforting position for the client. Figure 3-8 illustrates this positioning. Make sure the bed is level before a client moves into this position. If they can move on

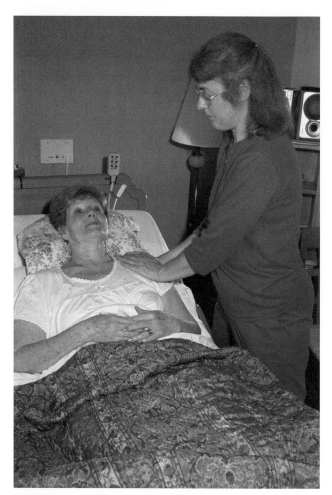

FIGURE 3-5. Client in hospital bed. The head of the bed has been elevated to accommodate the comfort of the client. Notice that the side rails have been lowered. If they are up before the Comfort Touch session, they must be returned to that position following the session.

their own, you can help provide support in positioning, but do not attempt to move the client by yourself. A pillow is placed under the head, ensuring that the head is in alignment with the back. A pillow is placed between the legs, to ease strain on the low back and hip. The client may hug a pillow for support. Sometimes a small towel is placed under the waist if support is needed there.

Variations on the Side-Lying Position

Variations to the basic side-lying position may be adopted, according to the needs and preferences of the client. The client may roll *forward* onto a soft pillow toward more of a prone position. Or she or he may roll *backward* onto a pillow toward a more supine position. The legs can both be bent at the knees, or one may be straight, the other bent. Any of these variations arise

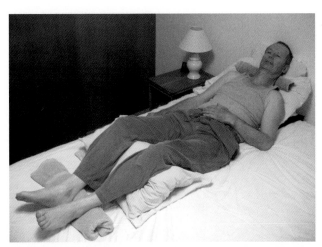

FIGURE 3-6. Client in standard double bed. Notice the use of pillows (minimum 2–3) to elevate the upper body. A neck roll made of a small towel is optional and is used if the pillows available are not soft enough to comfortably support the curve of the client's neck. Pillows are used to elevate the knees. This relieves stress on the lower back, prevents hyperextension of the knees and helps to relax the legs. Another option is to use a small towel that can be rolled and placed under the ankles. This prevents the heels of the client from rubbing on the bed, causing discomfort or pressure sores.

from the client's own particular situation. Notice what seems natural and comfortable to clients, making suggestions to enhance their comfort. With this population, it is usual to only have patients lie on one side only—the side of their choice—rather than rolling from one side to the other.

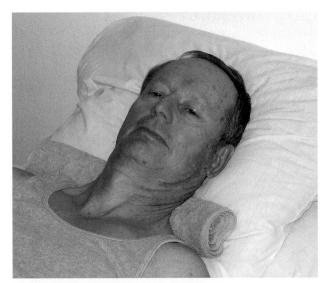

FIGURE 3-7. Neck support. A small towel can be rolled to support the neck. Check with the client for feedback and make sure it is not too thick.

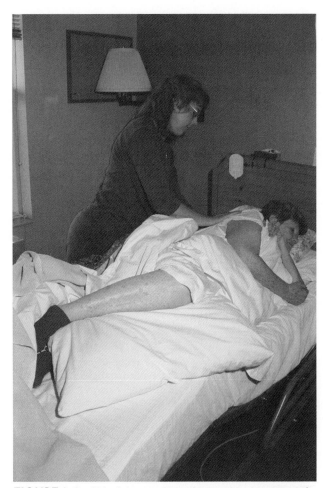

FIGURE 3-8. Side-lying position. Notice the placement of the pillows in the side-lying position. There is a pillow under the client's head, while another is placed between her legs to support the hips in a neutral position and provide cushioning between the bony surfaces of the knees and ankles. The client leans into or hugs a third pillow placed in the front of her chest.

Wheelchair

Use of the wheelchair for Comfort Touch offers a number of advantages. It allows the client to remain where they are during the day, without the logistical challenges of moving to a bed. The seated position allows him or her to breathe fully and deeply, as it opens up the respiratory passages. In the seated position the therapist is able to assess the posture of the client and facilitate a more erect and life-affirming posture. In the seated position, as shown in Figure 3-9, it is easy to work on the client's shoulders.

Always lock the brakes on the wheels of the chair when working, and make sure that the footrests are in a comfortable position for the client. With a client in the seated position, either in a wheelchair or a regular chair, place a towel over the back of a chair to support the client's upright posture. This also allows the therapist to

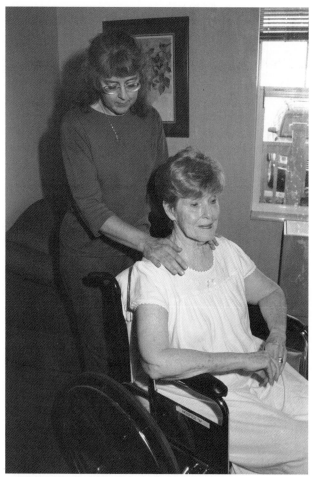

FIGURE 3-9. Seated position in a wheelchair. With the client seated in a wheelchair, it is easy to work on the shoulders, arms, and hands. A towel is placed over the back of the chair to give the client additional support and to facilitate a relaxed upright posture. Towels can also be placed on the armrests of the chair to pad the client's arms; or the armrests can be removed during a session, making it easier to access the arms and hands of the client.

use the back of the chair for leverage in applying pressure to the back, using various techniques of Comfort Touch, including *contact pressure,* along the erector spinae muscles on either side of the spine. In the seated position it is also easy to access the arms, hands, legs, and feet of the client.

Recliner

Many elderly people and those with limited mobility have reclining chairs that are comfortable to them. The use of these familiar chairs for Comfort Touch sessions offers all the advantages stated above for the seated position. Additionally, the clients have the extended back of the chair on which to rest their heads. The

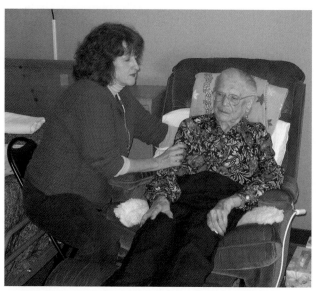

FIGURE 3-10. Seated position in recliner. The therapist sits beside her client and is able to reach under the client's upper back and shoulder to exert pressure there, using the back of the recliner for leverage. She can also work on the arms and hands of the client.

woman in Figure 3-10 receives the benefits of Comfort Touch while sitting in her own recliner. The therapist is able to sit beside her and reach the client's upper back and shoulder. She can also work on the arms and hands of the client.

While sitting in a recliner, the client's legs can rest on the elevated leg lift, and the whole chair can be adjusted to accommodate the client in a supine position. Occasionally, an additional pillow or towel may be used to facilitate the greatest resting position for the client. The therapist in Figure 3-11 gives a comforting foot massage to the client in her recliner.

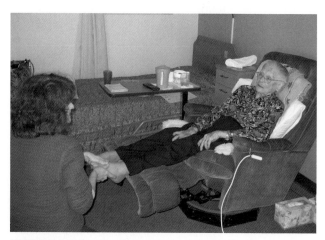

FIGURE 3-11. Foot massage in recliner. The therapist gives a comforting foot massage to the client in her recliner.

Generally, Comfort Touch is practiced with the patient using one of the above options for positioning, but there are times where the use of a massage table is appropriate. If so, be sure that the table is set to a low enough height that the client can get onto it without difficulty. If this is lower than the customary height at which you work on a table, you can use a stool and sit for more of the session. The recommendations for working supine on a bed apply, with ample use of pillows under the upper body and beneath the knees.

Remember that the elderly or those with various medical conditions may easily become dizzy or disoriented upon sitting up after lying supine. *Do not leave the elderly or fragile client alone to get on or off the table.* For liability reasons, some medical organizations (eg, hospice or home care) do not allow the use of massage tables for their patients. If a patient associates Comfort Touch of massage therapy only with the use of a massage table, they might think that they will not be able to receive this bodywork if they can't get on a table. Therefore, for the frail individual it is generally best to avoid using a massage table in favor of the other options discussed above in this section.

Body Patterning for the Practitioner

While it is important to ensure the safety and comfort of the client, the practitioner of Comfort Touch must also be attentive to one's own safety and comfort. The therapist needs to use good principles of biomechanics to be most effective in her or his work. Pay attention to your patterns of movement as you approach this work. Because working with the elderly and the ill requires adapting to the special needs of the client, it can take real flexibility and creativity to find comfortable ways of using your body as you touch the client.

Remember that it is *not* required to put yourself in an awkward or uncomfortable position to do this work. If you are uncomfortable, chances are that the client will sense your discomfort. Rather, you need to find different ways of using your body along with the use of helpful props, such as a stool or chair.

The following are some tips on body patterning.

Appropriate Clothing and Accessories

While clothing should be clean and professional-looking, it also needs to be comfortable, so that you can maneuver easily around the client and her or his chair or bed. Sometimes, you may need to sit on the bed or on the floor, so it is helpful to wear shoes that you can easily slip off. Before beginning a session, remove your wristwatch and jewelry from your hands and fingers. You may even want to change into clean socks, to ensure safety and proper hygiene for you and your client.

Spinal Alignment

Before you begin the hands-on work, be mindful of your own posture. Throughout the session, maintain awareness of proper spinal alignment. Balancing one major body mass over another, keep the head and shoulders upright and supported by your back, which in turn should rest on your pelvis, and your pelvis is on your legs. Don't strain forward with the head and neck or slump over the client's bed. Avoid bending and twisting your back.

Awareness of Breathing

Full, deep breathing helps you to be aware of your body, assisting you to sense instinctively how to move or position yourself in a healthy way. Full, relaxed breathing opens up your chest and abdomen, contributing to healthy spinal alignment. Ask yourself, "Am I comfortable? What could I do to get more comfortable?"

Get Close to the Client

Stand close to the client, or sit on a stool or chair placed close to the bed as you work, as shown in Figure 3-12. Avoid reaching too far out from your center of gravity, as your unsupported arms will tire quickly. Sometimes, you may sit on the bed itself, as illustrated in Figure 3-13. Before sitting on the bed, first check to make sure that it is okay with the client. If it does not seem appropriate to

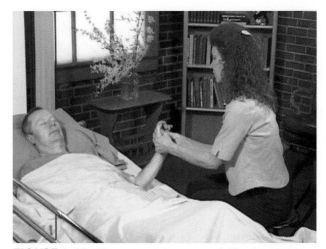

FIGURE 3-12. Therapist sitting on stool. The therapist sits on the folding metal stool in order to get close to the patient's bed. From this position she is able to press into the palm of the patient's hand.

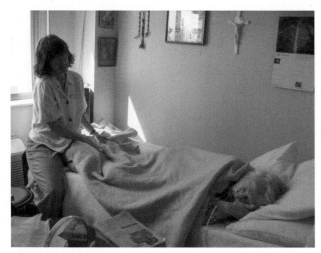

FIGURE 3-13. Massage therapist sits on bed. The therapist is sitting comfortably on the edge of the bed as she massages the patient's feet.

sit on the bed, simply work on the parts of the client's body that are most accessible. Or you may use the bed (or the wheelchair) to your advantage as you lean against it and let it support you. Be careful that you do not bump or jiggle the bed.

Move Slowly

Allow yourself time to move from one position to the next. It may take some time to ensure comfortable positioning of your client, as well as to figure out comfortable patterning for yourself. Moving slowly contributes to the atmosphere of safety and relaxation for the client.

Begin Where Access to the Client's Body Is the Easiest

Begin the hands-on session by working on the most accessible part of the client's body, usually the hands, the arms, or the feet. Approach the client from the side that is easiest to reach. This gives the client a chance to get familiar and comfortable with your touch. You can sit on a chair or stool to massage one hand, and then sit on the bed to massage the other hand. To work on the feet, sit at the foot of the bed, on a stool, or on the floor.

Face the Direction of your Work

If you are standing, face your client and step forward. One foot will be in front of the other in a relaxed and naturally aligned base of support. Movement educator Mary Ann Foster refers to this natural alignment of the body in performing massage as the "human stance."[1] From this stance, you can gently rock forward over your base of support, in the same way that you rock forward to take a step.

When you are sitting, lean forward from your base of support. Your hips and buttocks press into the seat of the stool and your feet press into the floor, as they would if you were standing. You can rock at the hips. Note that even as you are sitting, you will be most comfortable and effective if one foot is placed ahead of the other, rather than side to side. This patterning prevents strain to the low back.

If occasionally you are unable to face your hands and need to twist, make sure to lightly contract the deep lower abdominal muscles to stabilize your back and protect it from rotational injuries.

Press Through Your Feet As You Press Through Your Hands

When pressing into the client's body, also press into your own feet. This distributes the compressive forces through the core of your body, preventing strain and injury to the wrists and hands. Because this is a very cohesive and efficient way to use your body, it also gives an even, consistent, comforting pressure to the client. This awareness of your feet also keeps you grounded and focused, more fully aware of your own body, even as you pay attention to the needs of the client.

Keep the Wrists in a Neutral Position

Avoid sharp angles in the wrists and let your arms and hands extend naturally in from of you. You can imagine the energy of the earth coming up into your body from the soles of your feet, rising up through your torso, and radiating out through your hands.

Maintain a Natural Fluid Posture

Feel free to move your body as you work. Take advantage of the body's natural tendency to move in a subtle rocking motion which allows the body to continually rebalance itself around its vertical axis. By giving massage from a dynamic postural sway, both our movements and touch are more fluid and relaxed and our clients can feel the difference.[1]

The offering of Comfort Touch becomes a gentle dance as connection is made between the therapist and the client. Enjoy the subtlety of movement and easy exchange of energy. As you touch and press into each part of the client's body, feel the fullness of that part of the body as it returns into your hands.

Considerations Regarding Clothing and Draping

The techniques of Comfort Touch are based on the use of direct broad pressure and contact, so they do not require the use of lotions or oils on the skin. This simplifies the issue of clothing and draping, which is customary when offering the gliding and kneading strokes of conventional Swedish massage. For a Comfort Touch session the client can be fully clothed or dressed to their level of comfort. This also simplifies the logistics before beginning a massage with someone who has limited mobility. For this work the client may be wearing pajamas, a nightgown, or other comfortable clothes.

Sheets and blankets are still used, however, to ensure warmth and comfort for the client. Some clients will prefer to wear less clothing, in which case the sheet is also used to ensure modesty, as in conventional massage.

Use of Lotions and Oils

Massage oil or lotion is not necessary for most of the Comfort Touch techniques. Besides being unnecessary, there are specific reasons to avoid the use of these lubricants on the skin:

- **Petroleum-based oils.** Skin products which have a petroleum base (mineral oil) clog pores of the skin. One function of the skin is to eliminate wastes from the body, so it is important to keep the skin clean and free of barriers to this elimination. Skin care products may also have ingredients that can cause allergic reactions.
- **Vegetable-based oils.** These oils have limited shelf life, so they can become rancid. They are also difficult for the elderly or bedridden client to wash off. Preservatives and essential oils which are added to them can cause allergic reactions. They also tend to stain bed linens.

There are times when the use of a lotion or oil is appropriate. In these cases you may use an unscented moisturizing lotion or something that is familiar to the client:

- **Moisturize the skin.** Lotion can be used to moisturize the client's skin. This works well if the session is scheduled after a patient's bath time. Or you might use lotion on the hands and feet of the client, especially if the skin is dry. Remember that most Comfort Touch techniques do not require the use of lotion, so be careful when using lotion that you do not fall into familiar habits of using deep gliding strokes of conventional massage, which can tear or bruise the tissues.
- **Preference of client.** Some people enjoy the pleasurable sensation of having a good quality lotion smoothed on their skin. For the patient who is mostly clothed, lotion applied only to the hands and feet can satisfy this preference.

Ultimately, remember that the quality of touch is more important than any lubricant used. Many massage therapists find that when they don't use oil or lotion, or use it sparingly, it forces them to slow down and really connect with the client.

Listening and Adjusting to the Client's Needs and Feedback

Communication during the session follows the tone and intention established before beginning the hands-on work. You will continue to ask for the client's feedback throughout the session. This is especially important on the first visit while you establish rapport and adjust to the needs of this individual. You may need to restate that "This should be comfortable. If anything I am doing is uncomfortable please let me know." *Do not assume that you know how the patient feels.*

Here is a tip to help you in getting honest feedback from your clients. Instead of asking an open-ended question such as, "Is this okay?" or "How does this feel?" ask "What do you prefer—this amount of pressure? or this amount of pressure?" The first questions usually elicit a response of "It's okay," or "fine," leaving you unsure if the individual really is satisfied. The question, "What do you prefer—this? or this?" gives clients permission to be more specific in their feedback. It gives them a choice and helps them to feel in control.

Experiment with different ways of asking for feedback, as many people are hesitant to sound critical. They may be used to receiving unpleasant medical treatments and need assurance that this touch is meant to feel pleasurable, and that they are in control of what feels right for them.

Comfort Touch involves the knowledge and practice of a range of skills, guided by specific principles. It is also an art that makes use of the practitioner's intelligence, intuition, and creativity in adapting to an individual's needs. Remember that intuition involves full use of your senses, as you make decisions and adjustments based on the messages coming via those senses. Nonverbal communication is as important as verbal communication. Notice other ways in which people convey pleasure or displeasure with your touch. Use all your senses as you pay attention to the following clues:

- **What do you *see*?** Does the client grimace, or furrow her or his brows, or look away?
- **What do you *feel*?** Does the client flinch or tense up as you apply too much pressure? Do you feel her or him pull away?
- **What do you *hear*?** Does the client's breath change? Does she or he make sighs or moans indicating satisfaction, or other sounds indicating displeasure?

Whether through touch, words, or intention, effective communication involves a genuine desire to connect with the other person. Touch itself is a form of communication and affords a special opportunity to convey caring and compassion. As one elderly woman stated while receiving Comfort Touch, "This feels like communication."

Length of Session

All of the time you spend with a client is important. Maintain a respectful attitude when you are setting up before the massage, as well as after the session. The hands-on part of the session may be 30 to 50 minutes long, depending on the condition of the client and the feedback you receive. *Never work more than 1 hour.* Working too long can be too stimulating, or even tiring for the client. Initially you may want to work a shorter time, especially if the client has never had massage before. This will give you the chance to assess the person's response to your touch in the following hours and days.

If your time is limited, even 10 to 15 minutes can be beneficial. If you are the primary caregiver, or a nurse or nurse's aid, know that just a few minutes of comforting touch during the course of your other work can truly make a difference in the client's day.

STORY

Make Someone Happy

"Hello, Gracie. My name is Mary Rose. I am the massage therapist here," I said, introducing myself to the 93-year-old woman as she sat on the couch in the hospice care center where she was a patient. Sitting down beside her, I looked in her bright blue eyes, and took her hand in mine, as I said, "Would you be interested in receiving some Comfort Touch?"

Without objecting to the fact that I was holding her hand and gently touching her shoulder, she said, "Well, no. I don't believe in that stuff. I come from a medical family. My father was a doctor and we just don't go for that sort of thing." Still she seemed comfortable with my touch and leaned ever so slightly closer to me as I gently squeezed her shoulder, arm, and hand.

She continued to talk, chatting easily and commenting about the good care she was receiving in the care center. I held her hand for another moment between my hands and said, "Well, okay, Gracie, I'll be on my way now. You take care." She was smiling as I left the room.

A week later, I visited Gracie, introducing myself again. This time I had a student massage therapist with me whom I also introduced to her. Gracie said to me, "You look familiar. Don't I know you?" As I answered that I was the massage therapist, I took her left hand in mine. She said, "Oh my—your hands are so warm!" I affirmed that her hand did feel a little cold. So I continued to massage her hand, and then proceeded to using encompassing touch on her shoulder and arm.

"My other hand is cold, too," she said, as she offered me her right hand. So I repeated the Comfort Touch sequence on that side, as well. Taking my cue, the student spoke, "Gracie, would you like some Comfort Touch on your feet?" "Oh yes, they might be cold too." I continued to sit there as the student sat down on the floor and used encompassing contact pressure on her feet and lower legs.

"That feels good. I wonder what else on my body needs warming up!" Gracie exclaimed with delight. We both touched her a few more moments; then I said, "Gracie, we have to go now. Thank you for letting us spend this time with you."

She said. "Okay. You go and make someone else happy now."

After the Session

After the hands-on part of the session, you will want to pay attention to issues of closure and communication, safety concerns, and follow-up documentation.

Closure

Verbal communication and closure are very important aspects of the Comfort Touch session. While the words spoken can be simple, they do convey your caring and professionalism. For people coping with the challenges of age, infirmity, and terminal illness, simple kindness means a great deal. Offering massage within the hospice context particularly teaches you the importance of closure. For example, you learn that the time you have with clients may be your last. Your words of "goodbye" may be the last words they hear from you. The smile or look of contentment you see on their faces as you depart may be the last expression you see of them.

Close the hands-on part of the session in a gentle but deliberate manner that lets the client know that you are finished. You may hold your hands still for a few moments in the last position you touch. Then lift your hands a few inches away from the client's body, and hold for a few more moments before bringing your hands completely away. This allows a transition for the client from experiencing being touched to feeling the wholeness of her or his own body again.

This closing sequence can be accompanied by a few simple words that seem natural and appropriate. Examples include: "That's all for today." "Is there anything else you need before I go?" Or simply, "Thank you."

Safety

Before you leave, check with clients to see if they need anything rearranged to ensure their continued comfort and safety. You may need to adjust the pillows or linens on the bed. If you have elevated the height of a hospital bed, *be sure to lower it back to its previous lower level.* Return safety railings to their upright positions. Rearrange any furniture you may have moved, and take care that any medical equipment is safely in place and operating correctly. In some settings, there are foam pads that are placed on the floor beside the patient's bed for safety. Be sure they are in the proper place.

After the hands-on session, you will also want to thoroughly wash your hands and forearms again, using warm soapy water. Not only is this important from the standpoint of hygiene, but washing in warm water helps to relax your hands and arms, and gives you the opportunity to let go of the mental and emotional focus you held during the session.

Before leaving, check with the patients and/or their caregivers to make sure everything is okay. For example, you might check the room temperature again, or adjust a window opening or covering. Offer water to clients, and make sure they have personal items they need within easy reach, such as eyeglasses, a water glass, or tissues.

Communication and Documentation

Following the session, you will need to take a few minutes to write up your notes on the session. If you are in a facility, simply go to another room or waiting area to fill out your notes. If you have just visited a client at home, you can go sit in your car to document the session while it is still fresh in your mind. Use the CARE Note format detailed in Chapter 7. This system, compatible with the nursing documentation used in medical facilities, is easy to learn and use. Very simply, it asks the therapist to record the client's *condition* (C), the *action* taken (A), the client's *response* to the work (R), and her or his *evaluation* of the client's further needs for massage (E).

The first part of the CARE Note chart—the patient's condition—is a summary of the information you included in your intake form, with specific reference to her or his present condition. The action taken refers to the actual hands-on work you performed. The client's response refers to any noticeable reactions or physiolog-

ical responses to the work you did. The evaluation of the session is a place for you to record information that can help you in the next session in meeting the client's needs. It may also include any recommendation or information that may assist other caregivers of the patient.

Specific forms, like the sample in Chapter 7, can be used, or your charting can be written in narrative format within the nursing chart of the patient. This will depend on the policies and procedures of the setting within which you are working.

Proper documentation is important for the safety and well-being of the client. In a medical setting it allows communication between various caregivers of the patient. When visiting a patient in hospice or home care, you may be required to leave a phone message for the nursing case manager after each session. If there is information affecting the safety of the client, don't hesitate to call the patient's caregiver and share your observations with someone in charge. For example, report any bleeding, sudden changes in heart or respiratory rate, agitation, or complaints of pain by the patient. Sometimes the massage therapist is in a position to notice pressure sores, rashes, or bruises that may have been overlooked by others. If it is a serious situation, do not leave the patient until you know the issue has been addressed.

Remember the importance of confidentiality. Only authorized members of the patient's health care team should read the patient's chart. Do not share details of the patient's physical and mental condition, personal life, and family circumstance outside of the patient's authorized care team. CARE Notes need to be kept in a safe place out of view of all others. Follow your organization's rules about turning in notes to supervisors and/or disposing of outdated notes. Remember that a good therapeutic relationship is based on trust. The privacy of the patient and her or his family must be respected at all times.

Personal Growth and Change

Practicing massage with the elderly and the ill is a learning process. Over time you will hone your technical skills and become more comfortable with communication skills. It can be valuable to also keep a personal journal to record your thoughts, feelings, and questions. Different from a medical chart, this can be a place to focus on what you are learning and discovering as you do this work.

Practicing Comfort Touch, you have the opportunity to grow in compassion as an individual, meeting the challenges presented by association with those in need of your services. You have the opportunity to make a difference in the life of someone challenged by age, illness, injury, or loss. Your attitude, intention, and the skills you bring as you approach each session will be returned with gratitude as you make each person "feel like the most important person in the world."

Summary

- The roles and responsibilities of the Comfort Touch practitioners include adherence to the appropriate scope of practice of their profession; observance of specific protocols for hygiene; communication with clients and staff; and creation of a safe and healing environment.
- The Comfort Touch practitioner gathers pertinent information about the client prior to a session either directly from the client or indirectly through the client's caregivers. This includes the individual's contact information, a summary of her or his medical history and current health concerns, and a statement of their needs for Comfort Touch.
- While Comfort Touch techniques can be used even with the frailest client, there are precautions in the use of touch. For example, it is advised not to touch specific areas of tumors, sites of recent surgeries, inflammation, rashes, etc.
- The practitioner of Comfort Touch must be attentive to factors involving the safety or comfort of the client, paying attention to medical equipment, the positioning of the bed, temperature, lighting, etc.
- Comfort Touch is practiced with clients who may be in a standard bed, a hospital bed, a wheelchair, or a recliner. The supine, seated, and side-lying positions are used, according to the needs and preferences of the client. The prone position is avoided with this population.
- The practitioners of Comfort Touch must be attentive to their own safety and comfort, following the principles of biomechanics to be most effective in their work. This involves a number of factors including, but not limited to, awareness of spinal alignment, breathing, fluid movement, and body patterning in relation to the client.
- The practice of Comfort Touch is client-centered; therefore, the practitioner needs to be able to adjust to the client's needs and feedback, responding to verbal and non-verbal cues.
- Communication and documentation of a Comfort Touch session involves use of the CARE Note system of documentation. The therapist records the client's *condition* (C), the *action* taken (A), the client's *response* to the work (R), and *evaluation* of the client's further needs for massage (E).

Review Questions

1. Define *scope of practice*. What practices are included in a massage therapist's scope of practice? What practices are not?

2. What are the basic rules of hygiene for a massage therapist? What is the purpose of observing Universal Precautions?

3. Why is it important to observe rules of confidentiality?

4. Explain the concept of grounding.

5. What are the three primary components of a medical intake form?

6. List three tips for communicating effectively with the elderly and/or individual.

7. List five precautions in the use of touch.

8. Before beginning a Comfort Touch session, what are three of the factors that you need to address in order to create a safe and healing environment?

9. What is an advantage of the supine position for performing Comfort Touch? What is an advantage the seated position?

10. Explain three of the components of body patterning when practicing Comfort Touch. What do you anticipate to be your greatest challenges in doing this work?

11. Explain how you might evoke feedback from a Comfort Touch client? How do you respond to verbal and nonverbal feedback?

12. What are some important safety concerns to address after finishing the hands-on portion of a Comfort Touch session?

13. Why is it important to document the Comfort Touch session?

Reference

1. Foster MA. Your birthright: a case for the human stance. *Massage and Bodywork.* 2005;April/May:72–81.

Suggested Reading

Callahan M, Kelly P. *Final Gifts: Understanding the Special Awareness, Needs and Communications of the Dying.* New York: Bantam Books, 1993.

Centers for Disease Control and Prevention. *Standard Precautions: Excerpt from the Guideline for Isolation Precautions: Preventing Transmission of Infectious Agents in Healthcare Settings 2007.* http://www.cdc.gov/ncidod/dhqp/gl_isolation_standard.html. Accessed August 25, 2008.

Coulehan J, Block M. *The Medical Interview: Mastering Skills for Clinical Practice.* 3rd ed. Philadelphia: F. A. Davis; 1997.

Feil N. *The Validation Breakthrough: Simple Techniques for Communicating with People with "Alzheimer's-Type Dementia."* Baltimore: Health Professions Press; 1993.

Foster MA. *Somatic Patterning.* Longmont, CO: EMS Press; 2004.

MacDonald G. *Massage for the Hospital Patient and Medically Frail Client.* Baltimore, MD: Lippincott Williams & Wilkins; 2005.

Nelson D. *From the Heart Through the Hands: The Power of Touch in Caregiving.* Forres, Scotland: Findhorn Press; 2006.

4

The Principles of Comfort Touch: SCRIBE

OVERVIEW OF THE SIX GUIDING PRINCIPLES
OF COMFORT TOUCH: SCRIBE

SIX PRINCIPLES OF COMFORT TOUCH AND
HOW THEY RELATE TO TECHNIQUE

Slow
Comforting
Respectful
Into Center
Broad
Encompassing

> The river is flowing down to the sea
> O mother comfort me; your child I'll always be
> O mother carry me down to the sea.
> —From a song by Diana Hildebrand-Hull

*W*orking with the elderly or with people who are critically ill requires special sensitivity to their physical and emotional needs. On the one hand, Comfort Touch is very simple and instinctual—as natural as a mother's touch to comfort a child who is ill or has been injured. It arises from the basic human need to show care and concern for another human being who longs for connection. Yet many people lack the knowledge or confidence to offer touch that is safe, appropriate, and effective. Even the most experienced massage therapist or health professional can feel unsure about how to touch the medically fragile individual.

The style of massage known as Comfort Touch evolved out of the need to provide the benefits of touch to people whose physical conditions require an alternative to commonly practiced methods of massage. Techniques of conventional Swedish massage—effleurage, petrissage, vibration, friction, and tapotement—can be damaging to the fragile tissues of people of advanced age or infirmity. Most massage therapists learn the contraindications to the techniques they are taught for people with specific condition, but they do not learn how they *can* touch those people who are frail, elderly, or affected by chronic illness.

This chapter provides basic information to help the caregiver safely offer touch to those in need. It provides the following information:

- The six guiding principles of Comfort Touch.
- The relationship of these principles to the specific techniques of Comfort Touch.
- Exercises to assist practitioners of Comfort Touch to develop their awareness and understanding of these principles.

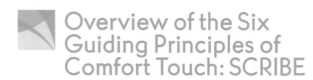

Overview of the Six Guiding Principles of Comfort Touch: SCRIBE

By following the guiding principles of Comfort Touch, the individual practitioner can apply the specific techniques of this style of bodywork with an understanding of their intention and purpose. There are six principles that form the foundation upon which to approach a session with a client. The word SCRIBE is used as a way to remember these principles.

The following words de*scribe* the general principles of Comfort Touch. Comfort Touch is:

- SLOW. The rhythm is slow, which creates a restful atmosphere. Pay attention to your own breath; let it be full and deep. Working at a slow pace allows you the opportunity to carefully assess in the moment what is safe and appropriate for the client, as well as to take care of your own body.

- COMFORTING. The intention is to offer comfort. Make the person comfortable and offer a soothing, comforting touch. Do not try to cure or fix the person. The word "comfort" literally means "with strength." To give comfort one must come from a place of inner personal strength and share that strength and support with the person who needs it.

- RESPECTFUL. Always maintain a respectful attitude toward your client, appreciating the vulnerability one may feel when being touched. A respectful attitude is compassionate and non-judgmental, and contributes to a safe and healing atmosphere. Be sensitive in every moment to the verbal and nonverbal feedback of the client.

- INTO CENTER. The direction of pressure in Comfort Touch is *in* to the center of the particular part of the body you are touching. Pressure is applied perpendicularly to the surface of the skin and layers of body tissues, thereby preventing tearing of the skin or bruising of the tissues. The focus of intention is *into* the core or central axis of the part of the body being touched. This specific direction of pressure and focusing inward of intention allows for a penetrating touch, even with light to moderate pressure. Both the giver and receiver of touch can experience a profound sense of connection.

- BROAD. In general, all strokes are applied with a broad, even pressure. This contributes to a feeling of soothing comfort and connection. While the pressure may be firm, the broadness of contact prevents the likelihood of injury or discomfort. Let the entire surface of your hand make uniform contact with the part of the client's body you are touching. Imagine that your hand is melting into the person's body.

- ENCOMPASSING. Let your touch surround the part of the person's body you are contacting. Be aware of the relationship between your two hands and the energetic field that exists between them. Hold the person in this space. Encompassing touch contributes to a feeling of wholeness, of being cared for, and being acknowledged as a worthwhile human being.

The principles of Comfort Touch also become a guide in your life as you let the meaning of each word influence your actions and attitudes throughout the day. These words can guide you to live a more meaningful life, mindful in each moment of the healing affect you exert on the world around you.

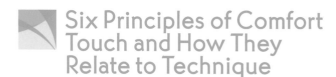

Six Principles of Comfort Touch and How They Relate to Technique

Let us explore these principles in greater depth and look at the rationales for their use. We will also see how they relate to the specific application of technique. Following the descriptions of each principle are experiential exercises designed to help the practitioner develop an understanding of the principle.

Slow

The first principle of Comfort Touch is *slow*. This principle is an important one to follow, because it contributes to the relaxing quality of the session and helps to establish an atmosphere of safety and trust. This refers to the rhythm and pace of the contact, but it also refers to the internal rhythm and quality of presence of the therapist.

Relaxing Quality of the Session

The techniques of Comfort Touch are practiced slowly, in a relaxed manner. In other styles of massage, by contrast, some techniques are done briskly. For example, some of the strokes of Swedish massage (petrissage, tapotement, vibration) can be performed quickly, with the intention of stimulating circulation or manipulating muscle tissues. But in this work, where the previously mentioned strokes are contraindicated, something else is required. The slowness of pace is calming and sedating to the client, and helps promote deep relaxation and relief from pain.

Safety and Trust

The slow pace of the work establishes an atmosphere of safety and trust. The therapist takes the time to tune into and carefully assess the needs of the client. The client does not feel overwhelmed or surprised with an unexpected touch. The slow pace at which the techniques are performed allows ample time for clear communication between the therapist and the client.

Rhythm of the Contact

While Comfort Touch is performed slowly, it is not static. There is a rhythm to this work. Think of the analogy of music. Generally, music that is played at a slower rhythm is more relaxing to the listener. When performing the specific techniques of *contact pressure* or *encompassing* (see Chapter 5), for example, each placement of the hands will be held for about 1 ½ seconds before moving on to the next placement. This slow, consistent pace imparts a trance-like quality, which is very sedating to the nervous system. While it has consistency, it also has variety. Like a well-crafted piece of music, there are moments of quicker tempo; for example, while gently pressing the palms of the hands or the fingers. There are also times to simply hold for several seconds; for example, while encompassing a joint like the shoulder or the knee.

The general rhythm established in this work is calming and comforting because of its sedating effect on the nervous system. This in turn affects the endocrine system, stimulating hormones which affect body chemistry and feelings of well-being. Studies have also been done that indicate that oxytocin is produced in the body in response to slow rhythmic touch.[1] Oxytocin is a hormone produced throughout the body but primarily in the pituitary gland, which, among other functions (eg, uterine contractions during childbirth), is associated with the phenomenon of bonding and feelings of connection.

Internal Rhythm of the Therapist

The living human body contains within it many rhythms operating throughout its various systems. These include the circulation of blood and lymph; the rhythm of the cerebrospinal fluid; the rates of digestion, metabolism, and respiration; the impulses of the nervous system; and the secretions from organs and glands. These separate yet interdependent internal rhythms operate without our conscious awareness, whether we are awake or asleep. However, we can also have an effect on these processes when we bring awareness to our breathing.

We can speed up or slow down our respiratory rate simply by bringing attention to it. When giving massage it can be very helpful to be conscious of the breath, inhaling and exhaling fully and deeply. This helps facilitate a sense of connection and relaxation within your own body, which in turn can be sensed by the client.

Exercise
CONSCIOUS BREATHING

Before beginning a session with a client, it is useful to take a few moments to become conscious of your own breathing. Conscious breathing is a way of *letting go* of your own physical discomforts or mental distractions and it is a way of *taking in* the life force necessary to nourish your body and enhance your sense of well-being.

To become aware of your breath:

1. Place your right hand on your abdomen, just below the navel, and let your belly expand as you inhale to allow for a deep and full breath.
2. Let the abdomen flatten as you relax and exhale.
3. Place your left hand on your upper chest over the sternum. Feel your ribcage expand and contract as you inhale and exhale.
4. Repeat several times.

You can practice this exercise anywhere, any time of the day. Even a breath or two taken consciously can shift your awareness and allow a change of perspective.

Exercise
CONNECT WITH A PARTNER'S BREATH

Practice this exercise with a partner, as you will be able to use it later when you work with a client. Have your partner sit in a straight-backed chair. You can place a folded towel behind her or his upper back to ensure that the back is in a straight posture.

1. Stand behind the person and place your hands on her or his shoulders. The palms should rest lightly on the thickest part of the trapezius muscle directly down below the ears.
2. Maintain this contact, noticing the movement in the body created by the person's inhalations and exhalations. Imagine that you are listening to the breath with the palms of your hands, lightening your contact with the inhalation and adding some pressure with the exhalation. (If you have difficulty feeling the movement created by your partner's breath, make sure that you are breathing fully yourself. Inevitably, this will allow you to feel the person's breath. It is *not* necessary to ask the person to take a breath.) Maintain this

connection through 3–4 cycles of the breath. The person being touched will realize, albeit subconsciously, that you are listening and paying attention to her or him in a profound way.

3. Bring your hands away from the person's shoulders, holding them about an inch away from the body. Hold this position through another cycle of her or his breathing, again noticing the movement in the body.

4. Bring your hands away and down to the side of your body.

This exercise provides an easy way to help someone to relax very quickly. It helps both the giver and receiver of touch breathe more efficiently, without the necessity of speaking or trying to manipulate the breath. It is a good way to begin a session of Comfort Touch with a client who is in the seated position, as seen in Figure 4-1.

Comforting

The second principle of Comfort Touch is *comforting*. It is the intention of this work to offer physical and emotional support through the use of proper positioning, appropriate techniques, and skillful communication. It is not the intention to try to fix, change, or cure the

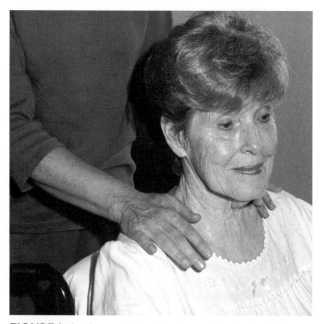

FIGURE 4-1. Connect with the client's breath. The therapist places her hands on the shoulders of the client. Having tuned into her own breath, she is able to tune into the breath of the client, feeling the subtle movement of her inhalations and exhalations. This allows the client to feel a sense of trust and connection with the therapist.

individual. Healing and change may occur, but that is secondary to the purpose of being present with the individual in the moment.

Definition of Comfort

The word *comfort* is derived from the Latin prefix *com,* meaning "with," and *fortis,* meaning "strong." Etymologically, the word *comfort* means to "make someone stronger," and its original English usage meant "to encourage or support." Through our touch we offer encouragement, helping people feel stronger in their ability to cope with the physical, mental, and emotional challenges they face.

Intention to Comfort

The intention of Comfort Touch is to offer comfort to enhance the quality of life for those in physical and/or emotional pain, discomfort, or distress. This idea is consistent with the universal and ancient traditions of healing by which the caregiver offers nurturing to the one in need. It is *not* necessary to try to fix or change the person. To give comfort one must come from a place of inner personal strength and share that strength and support with the person who needs it. The caregiver is *with* the client, supporting them where they are, physically and emotionally. The way in which touch is offered is assuring to the client, and provides a calming cloak of comfort. The client who is suffering with stress and discomfort can experience this influence as a welcome and soothing balm for her or his pain. Comfort *is* the antidote to discomfort.

The intention to comfort is also consistent with the basic premises of **palliative** medicine, which emphasizes the alleviation of symptoms without curing the underlying cause. In this growing medical specialty, health care providers—including physicians and nursing staff—strive to alleviate the severity of symptoms, thereby helping to improve the overall quality of life for people suffering with injury or illness. While this discipline grew out of the hospice movement and its work with the terminally ill, it has now expanded to include patients with serious chronic medical conditions, and can be seen as part of an integrated approach to medical care.[2] The practitioner of Comfort Touch can be seen as a complementary part of the health care team in the practice of palliative medicine.

Occasionally, otherwise well-meaning therapists or caregivers have the misguided notion that they are present to effect a cure for the one who is seriously ill, or—in the extreme—that they are sent on a mission "to assist the patient to die." In other words, they have an agenda. This is *not* the purpose of Comfort Touch. It is truly humbling to do this work—to be with people in what is often their most vulnerable time of life. But we cannot presume to know the outcome of someone's illness.

We are truly most helpful when we let go of our own agendas and offer support to people as they are. And yes, as we offer the gift of touch without concern for results, things can and do change. But it is not up us to become attached to how that change should look. Often the greatest healing comes when we let go of concepts about outcomes, and enjoy the interaction and experience in the present moment.

Make the Client Comfortable

Position the client to optimize her or his comfort. In working with those who are elderly or medically fragile, it is the job of the therapist to adapt to the clients' situations and ensure that they are in the most comfortable positions possible. Whether they are in a wheelchair, hospital bed, recliner, or regular bed at home, the therapist learns to figure out how to make them most comfortable. It is *not* necessary, or even desirable, to transfer the client to a massage table to offer Comfort Touch effectively. Make generous use of pillows and/or towels to help support the individual (Figure 4-2).

The Therapist Should Be Comfortable

When practicing Comfort Touch it is important that the therapist also be comfortable. The individual receiving touch will feel it—whether consciously or unconsciously—if the therapist is uncomfortable or in a compromising position. The therapist must use good body patterning, and can often benefit by using small stools and/or chairs to get into a comfortable position.

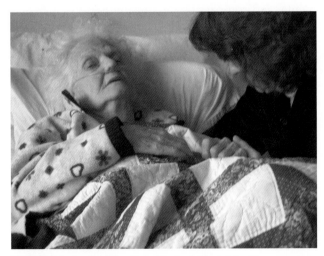

FIGURE 4-2. Position the client comfortably. The caregiver adjusts the position of the bed and the pillows and bedding before beginning the Comfort Touch session.

Comfort and Communication

The client will be comforted as you follow the guidelines offered through these principles and use the specific techniques of Comfort Touch. But your care and concern are also conveyed through the words you speak and the tone of voice you use. One client put it this way: "It's always so comforting to hear your voice." You can speak your intention to the client by saying, "I'm here to offer comfort. Let me know how I can help you."

Use words that acknowledge the experience of the client. "Yes, I understand that you are in pain." "Let me know what is helpful to you." To comfort also means to acknowledge the individual's inner strengths and resources. Speak in a manner that is uplifting. Just as the touch itself offers a pleasurable alternative to discomfort, so can your words. Sometimes it can be helpful to speak of something that is pleasant or meaningful to the individual. For example, it can be cheering to mention the beauty of a flower or some object in the room, or a blue sky that can be seen from the window. You might comment on a photo the client has in the room of a loved one.

Exercise
AWARENESS OF COMFORT

You may have a friend read this exercise to you, taking ample time after each question. Or you may do it by yourself, reading each question one at a time, tuning in for the answer to each question, and then writing it down.

1. Sit comfortably on a chair or lie on a mat on the floor, letting your body rest into your chosen position. Let your breath be full and deep.
2. Picture yourself as a child and remember a time that you were hurt or ill, and someone came to comfort you. What did you feel?
3. How did this person comfort you? Did she or he touch you? Did she or he speak? Did she or he offer something to you (eg, food, warmth)?
4. What happened after you were comforted? Did anything change? What was most helpful? What would have made it a better experience? For what were you most grateful?
5. Now remember a time when you were hurt—physically or emotionally—and no one was there to comfort you. What did you feel? What did you want or need?
6. Picture that situation now and imagine that someone comes to comfort you. Let yourself be comforted. Who comes? How does she or he comfort you? Does she or he touch you? Does she or he speak? Does she or he give you anything?

7. What happened after you were comforted? Did anything change? What was most helpful? What would make it a better experience? For what are you most grateful?

Take note of your experiences with this exercise. What does it tell you about how you like to be comforted? Do you want to be touched? If so, how do you want to be touched? Do you want to be spoken to? Do you resist being comforted? You can repeat this exercise, tuning into any part of your life, whether it be a physical or emotional trauma or discomfort. How do you comfort yourself?

Exercise
GETTING COMFORTABLE

Practice this exercise with a partner. You will need a flat surface—a bed, massage table, or mat on the floor. You will also need a variety of pillows, towels, and a blanket.

1. Have your partner lie down on her back. Notice if she appears to be comfortable to you. Ask her if she is comfortable, and let your partner make any necessary adjustments in positioning.
2. Next, offer her the option of having a pillow under her knees. Ask "Is this more comfortable or less comfortable?"
3. Try several other options: a pillow under the head; a rolled up hand towel under the head; pillows or towels under the arms; a blanket for added warmth; the repositioning of the legs or arms; dimming the lights; playing or adjusting the volume of music. With each option, ask, "Is this more comfortable or less comfortable?"

Often people will say they are comfortable, but when given more options, they discover something that is *more* comfortable for them. This is especially true of someone who is suffering from illness or is bedridden. For example, people who have difficulty breathing may be much more comfortable if their heads and backs are elevated in an incline using two or three pillows. Repeat the previous exercise with your partner in the side-lying position.

Exercise
INTENTION OF COMFORT

This exercise is practiced with three people. One person, "A," sits in a chair or lies down. The other two people will be touching "A." Out of earshot of the "A," they will agree to play one of two roles: "B" will touch the person with the intention of fixing her problem or curing the symptom. "C" will touch the person with the intention to offer comfort. Do not convey this to "A," but take turns touching this client staying with your agreed upon intention.

1. Before you touch "A," ask if there is anything bothering her that may need attention. Does she have a particular area of pain or discomfort?
2. Taking her words into consideration, proceed to touch her while staying with your agreed upon intention. "B" or "C" will work for several minutes, followed by the other. You may repeat.
3. Have "A" report on the experience. What did "A" notice as "B" worked on her? What did "A" notice when "C" worked on her?

You can all take turns playing the roles of "A," "B," or "C." Talk about your experiences. What did you learn? Did you have a preference? Might the intention of "B" or "C" be appropriate in different contexts or at different times?

You can do this exercise using the techniques of Comfort Touch or any other technique, with the intention being the variable.

Respectful

The third principle of Comfort Touch is *respectful,* which characterizes the attitude one maintains when offering touch. An attitude of respect allows the client to feel honored, and acknowledges the uniqueness and wholeness of the person. Your manner should be nonjudgmental and compassionate, contributing to a safe and healing atmosphere for the client.

Definition of Respect

The word *respect* is derived from the Latin prefix *re* meaning "again" and *spec,* meaning "look." Therefore, the word *respect* literally means "to look again." When we have a respectful attitude toward someone, we are free to "look again" in each moment as we interact with the person and not be limited by our first impressions. A respectful attitude conveys politeness, honor, and esteem.

Respect and Honor

When we touch another person, we are not merely touching a body; we are touching the person's mental and emotional reality as well. The experiences of a

Hints for Practice

Empathy

An important aspect of practicing Comfort Touch is attention to the positioning of the client, to ensure that he or she is in the most comfortable position possible. The options presented in Chapter 3 show you different ways of working with the client (eg, in the seated, supine, or side-lying positions), making the client more comfortable with the use of pillows and towels. But how do you know what is the best option for the client, or what options you might suggest to the client?

Here is what I do. I look at the client who is sitting in a wheelchair or recliner and ask myself, "Would I be comfortable sitting like that?" I imagine my body sitting in the same position as the client. For example, I notice that if my back were in that position, it would exaggerate the curvature of my thoracic spine, causing pain, and wonder to myself, "What could I do to alleviate that?" Upon reflection, I decide that a soft pillow or towel behind the back might help to support it to have better alignment, thereby easing the discomfort. So I try that with the client,

and ask, "Is this more comfortable or less comfortable?" and listen to the answer.

With a client who is lying supine, I notice the alignment of the spine. I imagine myself in that position, and ask myself, "Would <u>my</u> neck be comfortable or feel supported in that position?" or "How could <u>I</u> breathe in this position, if I had limitations to my breathing?" I can try placing a different pillow under the head and neck, or placing a small rolled up hand towel under the neck. Again, I ask the client, "Is this more comfortable or less comfortable?" and listen to the answer. I might notice the position of the client's legs, and ask "How would <u>my</u> knees or lower back feel in this position?" You can offer to place a pillow under the knees to flex the client's knee and hip joints, alleviating strain in the client's low back. Again, ask the client for feedback.

This process involves (1) observing the client, (2) imagining how it would feel in your own body, and (3) suggesting ways to make adjustments. It is a useful way to build empathy with the client. With practice, you will notice that you feel better in your own body as soon as you make adjustments for the client.

---

lifetime are recorded in the nervous system of the body. We contact that reservoir of sensation when we connect through touch, acknowledging the wholeness of one's being. One woman spoke these words after receiving Comfort Touch: "During that hour I felt like I was the most important person in the world." What a gift it is to let her know that she is important and deserving of respect and honor.

Healing is the process of creating and acknowledging the experience of wholeness. As practitioners of Comfort Touch it is not our intention to effect a cure with our clients; rather, we are involved in a process that respects the totality of the individual being. A healthy individual is not necessarily someone who is free of disease, but rather someone who knows she or he is whole, no matter what her or his immediate physical, mental, and emotional circumstances may be.

Nonjudgmental Attitude

We do not comfort people by judging them. A respectful attitude involves accepting people as they are, without criticizing them or blaming them for their circumstances. For example, if you touch someone who is ill, and you are thinking or saying, "What did you do

to create this situation for yourself?" you are blaming that individual for having the illness or injury. If the client internalizes that question, they might think, "What *did* I do? There must be something wrong or bad about me." The thoughts and questions may not even be conscious, but they may evoke uncomfortable feelings in the individual.

Here is another example: You begin to massage a person's shoulder and comment "Wow, you are really tight here! You need to let me work this out." You may be well-intentioned, but you might also be conveying the message, "You are not okay the way you are. I need to fix you." The client may even agree with you, but you have not empowered them. You are not comforting them. You may be reinforcing her or his self-judgment.

However, it is natural to notice what you will, and let your attention—and the client's—focus on the body part being touched. Rather than tell the person what you notice, you could ask, "What do *you* notice here?" It is okay to ask clients about their experience and solicit their feedback to your touch. This allows them to remain in control of their own experience. As your contact embraces the muscle, let it soften or release if it is ready.

Remember that the meaning of respect is "to look again." You may see the individual and form an opinion or judgment about them. In itself, that is not a problem. Most of us have the habit of forming judgments, but it is presumptuous to tell another person what she or he are experiencing. The important practice is simply to notice the judgment and release it. Look again.

A respectful, nonjudgmental attitude also contributes to a more satisfying experience for the therapist. Freed of the need to judge, analyze, or fix the client, therapists can focus their attention on being fully present with the client, allowing the power of touch to comfort in the moment, as illustrated in Figure 4-3.

A Place of Refuge

Your respectful attitude establishes an atmosphere of trust and creates a place of safety and refuge for the client. It is important to appreciate the vulnerability the individual may feel about being touched. Touch can evoke feelings of pleasure or pain. Touch can evoke memories, fears, longings, and/or curiosity. Pay attention to anything that might arise in the client's experience. Listen to what the client tells you, both verbally and nonverbally. Be sensitive to her or his feedback to your touch.

Exercise
LETTING GO

This is a practice to help you learn to feel at ease with the world around you. By practicing letting go of judgments and attachments, you become less controlled by them.

1. Sit comfortably and close your eyes. Begin to notice your breathing.

2. Do not try to change your breathing or do anything in particular. Simply continue to breathe, letting go of each exhalation. As you notice other bodily sensations or feelings, observe them and let them go, as if you were watching clouds pass by (Figure 4-4).

3. As thoughts come into awareness, observe them and let them go. Do not try to push them away; simply let them go.

4. If judgments come into awareness, observe them and let them go. You may notice judgments of yourself or judgments of others. Do not fight the thoughts that come; simply notice them and let them go.

Do this exercise for 10 minutes a day for 1 week and notice how it affects your life. You can also apply this awareness to your everyday life. For example, notice when a judgment comes into your mind during the day. See if you can let go of it. You may need to acknowledge the thought and dialogue with it for a while before letting it go.

It is helpful to cultivate a sense of humor. Do not take your thoughts too seriously. Remember the bumper sticker that says, "Don't believe everything you think."

Exercise
ENVISIONING A REFUGE

Practice this exercise with a partner, who will guide you through the visualization. Then trade places as you guide your partner. Afterwards, you can talk about your experiences. After your initial experi-

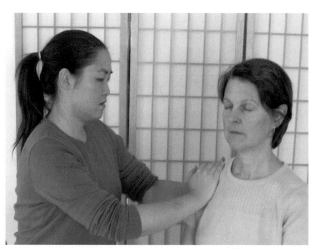

FIGURE 4-3. A respectful attitude. The therapist holds a respectful attitude toward her client, allowing the power of touch to comfort in the moment.

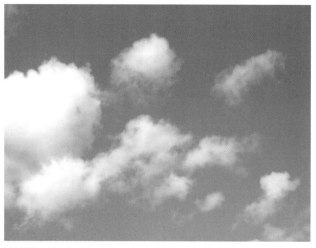

FIGURE 4-4. Letting go. Observe your thoughts and feelings, letting them go as if they are clouds in the sky.

ence, you can practice this exercise by yourself, imagining yourself in a safe and healing environment.

1. Sit comfortably and close your eyes. Let your breath be full and deep. Continue to notice your breath until you feel an easy, steady, effortless breath.
2. Picture in your mind's eye a place you would enjoy visiting. It can be somewhere that is familiar to you, or you can imagine a scene that is comforting and restful to you. Where is it? What does it look like? Is it outside in nature, or is it inside a building? What else do you notice about this place? Light? Colors? Objects? Smells? Temperature? People?
3. See yourself in this place of refuge. How does it affect you? How does your body feel as you let yourself be present in this scene for a few moments?
4. After a few minutes of visualizing and feeling yourself in this place, let the image dissolve. Return to the awareness of your body and your breath. Slowly open your eyes.

How do you feel when you bring your attention to your actual surroundings? Can you maintain the feeling that the place of refuge provided for you? When practicing Comfort Touch with a client, you can imagine that you are both in a place of refuge.

Into Center

The fourth principle of Comfort Touch is *into center*. This describes the direction of pressure the therapist applies relative to the surface of the body of the client. This awareness is key to the specific techniques of Comfort Touch. It describes a safe way to touch the person, as well as an effective way to bring the benefits of touch to those in need. The specific direction of pressure and focusing inward of intention allows for a penetrating touch, even with light to moderate pressure. Both the giver and receiver of touch experience a profoundly deep sense of connection.

Angle and Direction of Pressure

The direction of pressure in Comfort Touch is *in* to the center of the particular part of the body you are touching. Pressure is applied perpendicularly to the surface of the skin, thereby preventing tearing of the skin or bruising of the tissues. The focus of intention is into the central axis of the part of the body being touched. Apply firm, broad, even pressure to the area at a 90-degree angle from the surface of the skin. Slowly and deliberately, direct the pressure through the lay-

ers of body tissues into the center of the part of the body you are touching. Let the pressure of your contact *sink* into the center. Do not push. As you work slowly, you will tune into the client's body, feeling how much it will let you in. The arrows in Figure 4-5 indicate the angle and direction of pressure when touching the arm.

The phrase "into center" does *not* mean you are directing pressure toward the heart. This distinguishes it from some conventional massage strokes. If you are applying pressure correctly, there is no friction or pulling on the skin. This is one reason that lotions or oils are not required for this work. It is easy to tell if your angle of pressure is correct when you work through a client's clothing; if it is, you will not be wrinkling the fabric or pushing it in one direction or the other.

It is easy to picture the central axis of the arms and the legs, along with the fingers and toes. The anatomical center is the long bone around which the other layers form. When working on the head, the center is always

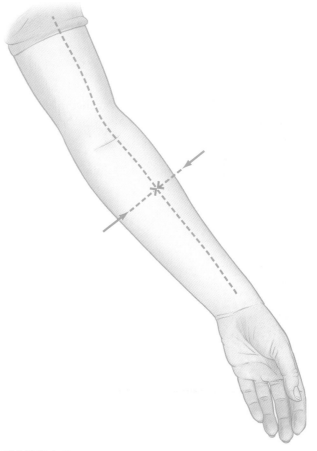

FIGURE 4-5. Into center of the arm. In the practice of Comfort Touch pressure is applied perpendicularly to the surface of the skin, and <u>in</u> to the central axis of the body part being touched.

somewhere near the center of the skull. It may be a little more confusing to think *into center* when touching the muscles of the shoulders or back. The arrow in Figure 4-6 indicates the direction of pressure into the belly of the upper trapezius muscle. Notice that the point of contact is still perpendicular to the skin and the direction of pressure goes through the layers of tissue toward the central axis of the body. The key thing to remember when applying pressure to the back is that your contact is perpendicular (90 degrees) to the surface of the skin, not pulling the skin at all. For example, as you press along the erector spinae muscles lateral to the spine, let your touch sink into and through the mass of those muscles.

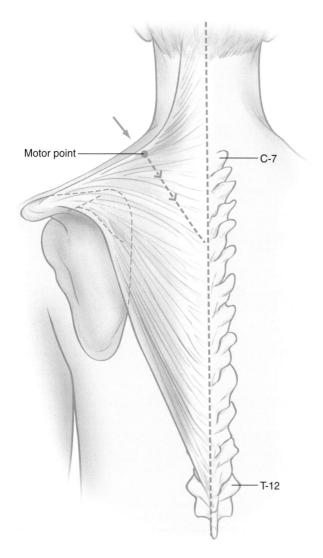

FIGURE 4-6. Into the motor point of the trapezius muscle.
This diagram shows the motor point in the belly of the upper trapezius muscle at the top of the shoulder. Access to the point is located below the ear and slightly posterior to the midline of the top of the shoulder. Pressure should be applied perpendicularly to the skin, and directed <u>in</u> to the central axis of the body.

Breaking Habits

If you are used to performing massage strokes which involve gliding, pushing, rubbing, or kneading, you will need to be especially careful to break the habit of doing them when offering Comfort Touch. With most common massage techniques, such as those just mentioned, it is easy to *see* what you are doing. With Comfort Touch techniques, applying pressure "into center," it is not so obvious to see what you are doing. You must be especially sensitive and pay attention in the moment. It is also important to receive this work by trading with a practice partner, so that you can learn and experience in your own body the practical application of this principle.

Benefits of Direct Pressure

The type of touch characterized in this principle of "into center" has specific benefits for the client:

- **Safety.** Because you are not creating friction on the skin, and because you are using a broad contact, there is minimal opportunity to tear the skin or underlying fragile tissues.
- **Sedating effect.** This work is sedating to the nervous system, because the focus and intention of the contact goes deep into the center of the part of the body being touched, calming the nervous system. In contrast, touch which only stays on the surface or rubs the surface is stimulating to the peripheral nerves, which can be irritating, ticklish, or even painful.
- **Respect for the integrity of the body.** When following this principle, you are respecting the integrity of the layers of body tissues. Start by contacting the surface of the skin. Next, allow your touch to affect the deeper layers of the skin. Continuing, let your touch sink into the superficial fascia (adipose layer), the deep fascia, the muscle layers, and, ultimately, the bone. This direct compression acknowledges the integrity of the layers, rather than separating or manipulating them, thereby contributing to a feeling of wholeness. See Figure 1-6.
- **Circulation.** Whereas the primary function of Comfort Touch is not to increase circulation of blood and lymph, it does, however, stimulate the flow of these fluids because of the alternating pressure and release. It does this at the same time as it is sedating the nervous system.
- **Perception of wholeness and connection.** Your touch conveys radiant warmth, felt by the client as you connect into her or his center. One individual described this as "a full and warm spaciousness . . . with much substance." It helps the client feels grounded and connected to one's core of being.

Exercise
GOING INTO THE CENTER THROUGH THE LAYERS

Before beginning this exercise, you may wish to review the anatomy of the part of the body you are touching (for example, the muscles of the upper leg, the quadriceps). In order to visualize tissue layers review Figure 1-6.

1. Sit comfortably in a chair. You may close your eyes. Place the palm of one of your hands on the surface of your thigh. Slowly begin to visualize the layers of this part of your thigh.
2. Notice the contact of your hand on the skin. Picture the deeper layers of the skin.
3. Continuing to hold the palm of your hand on the surface, let your hand sink into the next layer. Picture the superficial fascia (adipose layer) beneath the skin.
4. Let your pressure increase slightly as you picture the deep fascia, which surrounds the muscles.
   a. Continue with more pressure as you picture the layers of muscle, the quadriceps.
   b. Maintain a constant pressure as you picture the femur bone.
5. Release and repeat on another part of your body.

Notice as you do this exercise that your attention becomes focused as you allow time to sink through each layer of the body. You can also do this exercise without exerting pressure. Simply place your hand on the surface of the skin and imagine the layers, one by one.

Practice this exercise with a partner. Have one person lie down on a massage table. The partner then touches a part of the body (ie, the upper leg or arm) while visualizing the layers of body tissues. After taking turns, discuss your experience.

Exercise
GIVING/RECEIVING PRESSURE INTO CENTER

Practice this exercise with a partner. Let your partner sit in a chair.

1. Place a chair beside your partner and sit so that you are facing each other.
2. With your thumbs parallel and pointing upward, wrap your hands around your partner's upper arm.
3. Apply a broad, even pressure directly into the central axis of the arm, in toward the bone. (You can think of this as the even pressure that is applied with a blood pressure cuff.) Hold for a few seconds.
4. Let your partner give you feedback. Was the pressure even? Was it into the center?

Practice on other parts of the body, for example, the shoulders, the arms or the back. It is very important to practice this exercise with a partner, not only to practice *giving* pressure into the center, but also to experience how it feels to *receive* pressure into the center. Only when you comprehend the quality of touch that underlies this principle in your own body will you be able to fully convey that quality of touch to your clients.

Broad

The fifth principle of Comfort Touch is *broad.* In general, strokes of Comfort Touch are applied with a broad, even pressure. This contributes to a feeling of soothing comfort and connection. While the pressure may be firm, the broadness of contact prevents the likelihood of injury or discomfort. Let the entire surface of your hand make uniformly even contact with the part of the client's body you are touching. Imagine that your hand is melting into the person's body.

Broad, Full Hand Contact

In doing this work your hands are very relaxed, with minimal tension held in the ends of the fingers or thumbs. Your primary points of contact with the client's body are through the palms of your hands, with the digits gently wrapping or resting on the body. This approach conveys feelings of warmth and safety. As you touch different parts of the body, adjust your contact so that it is as broad as possible. The contact is not pushy, but it is deliberate and firm, thereby never pinching, poking, or tickling. Figure 4-7 demonstrates the use of broad, full hand contact on the back of the client.

Palms of the Hands

The palms of the hands, as well as the fingertips, contain specialized sense organs called tactile corpuscles, which are especially sensitive to pressure (see Figure 1-3). By bringing awareness to your palms as you touch the client, it is easy to sense and gauge the amount of pressure appropriate for that individual. You can "listen" with the palms of your hands as you exert pressure into the center of the part of the body you are touching.

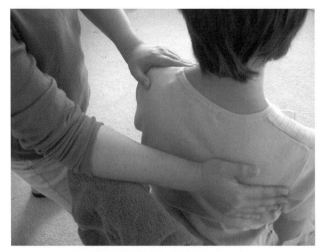

FIGURE 4-7. Broad full hand contact. The therapist applies broad, even pressure to the back of the client.

Exercise
FINGERTIP TOUCH VS BROAD TOUCH

Practice this exercise with a partner. Let your partner sit in a chair. Do this exercise in silence.

1. The partner who is sitting can close her or his eyes.
2. In succession touch five different parts of your partner's body lightly with your fingertips. For example, the top of the head, the right cheek, the left shoulder, a forearm, and a knee.
3. In succession touch five different parts of your partner's body lightly with the palm of your hand.
4. Repeat the first two steps, but touching with a firmer, deeper pressure.

Let the partner who is sitting give feedback on this experience. How did it feel to be touched lightly with the fingertips or lightly with the palm of the hand? How did it feel to be touched with a deeper fingertip pressure or a deeper pressure with the palm of the hand?

Trade roles and repeat the exercise.

Notice the quality of touch with the various types of contact. What is most relaxing or soothing? Think about how this might relate to the overall experience of being touched in a Comfort Touch session.

(Note: The exercise on *Shaping* in the next section also demonstrates the principle of "Broad.")

Encompassing

The sixth principle of Comfort Touch is *encompassing*. Let your touch surround the part of the body you are touching. Be aware of the space between your two hands. Hold the person in that space. While this principle describes techniques, it also describes an attitude. Encompassing touch contributes to a feeling of wholeness and connection. The giver of Comfort Touch holds a nurturing presence, which allows the client to feel cared for and acknowledged as a worthwhile human being.

Shaping

As you touch your client with both hands, let your hands conform to the shape of the part of the body you are touching. For example, as you hold the person's hand between your own, let your hands wrap around that hand, molding to its shape. Likewise, as you hold the person's arm, your hands wrap around the arm, applying an even, broad pressure as they conform to the shape of the arm, as shown in Figure 4-8.

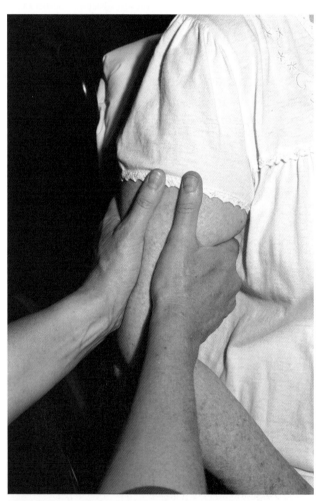

FIGURE 4-8. Encompassing the arm. The therapist's hands encompass and conform to the shape of the client's arm as they apply broad, even pressure. Notice that the thumbs are parallel. This ensures that the palms of the hands and the broader surfaces of the thumbs, rather than the thumbtips, exert an even pressure around the client's arm.

When touching a large area, such as the back, let your touch acknowledge the shapes and contours of the body. When touching a limb or a toe, encompass and enfold that part of the body. One client described it this way: "It is like receiving a hug to every part of the body." Encompassing touch conveys a feeling of acknowledgment, safety, and support.

Space and Substance Between Your Hands

The principle of encompassing describes a way of contacting the surface of the body you are touching with your hands. It also gives a way to think about the space *between* your hands and the substance you are holding in that space. For example, as your hands encompass a person's head, be aware of all that is contained between your hands. Think not only about the physical structures involved, but the tremendous life force contained and circulating within the body you are touching. See Figure 4-9.

held. Let it become the shape of the one it is holding. Release.
3. Touch another part of your body, "shaping" to that form. Release.
4. Maintaining a soft focus with your eyes, get up and walk around the room, touching various objects; for example, the door handle, a cup, a pencil, a book. If it is a small object, you can use one hand to conform to its shape. If it is a larger object it may require both hands to encompass it.
5. Notice the texture of the objects you touch, and how you adjust your contact to respect the material substance of the object. For example, you might grip a ceramic bowl firmly in both hands to hold it. In contrast, as you hold a flower in your hand, you would need to hold it carefully to avoid crushing it, as shown in Figure 4-10.

Exercise
SHAPING

1. Sit quietly for a few moments with your eyes closed.
2. Take one hand and hold it with the other hand. Let your holding hand form around the one being

Exercise
SHAPING WITH A PARTNER

1. Sit quietly with your eyes closed.
2. Have your partner hand you various objects, one at a time; for example, a rock, scissors, paper, a bowl, a feather.
3. Let both of your hands encompass each object, shaping your hand to the object. Maintain as broad a contact as possible.

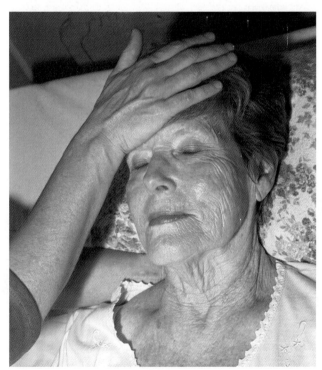

FIGURE 4-9. Encompassing the head. As the therapist encompasses the client's head, he or she is aware of all that is contained between the space of his or her hands.

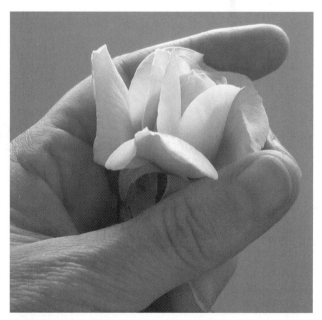

FIGURE 4-10. Shaping. Let your contact conform to the shape of the object you hold. As you encompass an object as delicate as this rose, you must be careful to avoid crushing it.

Remember this exercise when you are touching a client, letting your touch conform to the shape of the part of the body you are touching.

Exercise
SPACE BETWEEN THE HANDS

1. Sit in a chair with your feet flat on the floor. Let your breath be full and deep.
2. Hold your hands out in front of you, fingertips up and palms facing each other, a few inches apart. The hands should not be rigid.
3. Bring your hands as close together as you can without actually letting them touch. Be aware of the space between the fingertips and the palms of your opposing hands.
4. Let your hands move apart a few inches. Then bring them back together again, as close as possible without touching.
5. Continue this exercise, letting the hands move apart and together. Let them get close, then move apart to varying distances. Notice what you feel. Continue to breathe throughout.

What do you notice? Heat? Pressure? Other sensations? Nothing? There is no right or wrong way to do this exercise, and different people may experience different sensations when practicing it. Try it on different days, and see if you have a different experience each time. Notice how sensations may vary with the hands at varying distances apart.

Some people experience the space between their hands as a magnetic field with sensations of pressure or resistance. Indeed, the human body is surrounded and infused by electromagnetic fields. This exercise can bring your attention to this phenomenon. Others may attribute the sensations simply to the warmth of the hands themselves, and the ability to sense the conduction of heat.

When applying this awareness to the techniques of Comfort Touch, it is useful to realize that the space between your hands is important relative to touch. As you focus your attention on the space between your hands, you intensify the experience of the field between them. When you touch someone with your hands, you are allowing them to rest in the space, warmth, and energy between your hands.

Summary

- There are six principles that guide the practice of Comfort Touch. These principles inform the rhythm, intention, attitude, and techniques of this modality of bodywork.
- The word SCRIBE is used as a way to organize and remember these principles, which are *slow, comforting, respectful, into center, broad,* and *encompassing.*
- The rhythm of Comfort Touch is *slow.* Working at a slow pace creates a restful atmosphere for both the giver and receiver of touch.
- The intention of Comfort Touch is *comforting.* Emphasis is placed on making the person comfortable and using techniques that are comforting to the per-

son. The practitioner is not concerned about fixing, curing, or changing the person.

- The practitioner of Comfort Touch maintains a *respectful* attitude toward the client. A respectful attitude is compassionate and nonjudgmental, and contributes to a safe and healing atmosphere.

- The direction of pressure in Comfort Touch is *into* the *center* of the part of the body being touched. Pressure is applied perpendicularly to the surface of the skin and layers of body tissues, thereby preventing tearing of the skin or bruising of the tissues. This specific direction of pressure and focusing *into center* allows for a penetrating touch that is calming and sedating to the nervous system of the client.

- In general, strokes are applied with a *broad*, even pressure, with emphasis on contacting the client with full contact of the palmar surfaces of the hands. This contributes to a feeling of soothing comfort and connection.

- Techniques of Comfort Touch provide *encompassing* contact to the part of the client's body being touched. Encompassing touch contributes to a feeling of wholeness and safety.

- The principles of Comfort Touch also become a guide in your life as you let the meaning of each word influence your actions and attitudes throughout the day. These words can guide you to live a more meaningful life, mindful in each moment of the healing affect you exert on the world around you.

 ## Review Questions

1. What are the six principles of Comfort Touch?
2. Which principle describes the rhythm of Comfort Touch?
3. Describe the primary intention of Comfort Touch.
4. Why is a nonjudgmental attitude important to the practice of Comfort Touch?
5. What characterizes the direction of pressure in Comfort Touch?
6. How is pressure applied in Comfort Touch? Explain the function of the tactile corpuscles in the palms of the hands.
7. How does the principle of *encompassing* relate to both technique and attitude when practicing Comfort Touch?

References

1. Angier N. *Woman: An Intimate Geography.* New York: Houghton Mifflin; 1999.
2. Pan CX. Palliative Medicine. *ACP Medicine Online.* http://www.acpmedicine.com/LandingPages/med0009.htm. Accessed August 12, 2008.

Suggested Reading

Rose M. *Comfort Touch—Massage for the Elderly and the Ill* [videotape and video guide]. Boulder, CO: Wild Rose; 2004.
Smith I. *Providing Massage in Hospice Care: An Everflowing Resource.* San Francisco, CA: Everflowing; 2007.

Techniques of Comfort Touch

> Become the practitioner you would want to go to if you were sick.
>
> —J. R. Worsley

Learning the techniques of Comfort Touch follows naturally upon familiarizing yourself with the principles that provide the foundation for this modality (SCRIBE). These techniques do not require the use of lotion, so they can be practiced on the individual who is fully clothed, or dressed according to her or his own comfort. After initial intake with the client, you will begin the session by making her or him comfortable in the position that is most appropriate, making use of pillows for support where necessary.

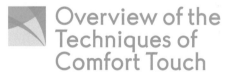

Overview of the Techniques of Comfort Touch

The techniques of Comfort Touch follow the guiding principles described in Chapter 4. After *slowing* down to connect with the client, the practitioner holds the intention to offer *comfort*, with an attitude that is *respectful* of the person being touched. The direction of pressure is *into the center* of the part of the body being touched, with *broad, encompassing* contact. The exercises from the previous chapter are useful in the exploration of the meaning of these principles.

While there is an apparent simplicity to this work, the practitioner of Comfort Touch will discover deeper layers of intricacy as the techniques are applied to each individual. It is important that the techniques of Comfort Touch be practiced accurately for greatest effectiveness. Comfort Touch is *not* a light form of conventional Swedish massage. It does *not* use effleurage, petrissage, or kneading where these strokes can damage the tissue of the person whose body is compromised by age or ill health. More importantly, Comfort Touch acts on the nervous system in such a way that it causes deep relaxation by calming and sedating it, which also accounts for its effectiveness in relieving pain. There are many specific techniques that can be used in this work, depending upon the condition of the client and the training and skill level of the practitioner.

Awareness of Anatomy

The study of anatomy enhances the quality of Comfort Touch by helping the therapist to visualize and appreciate what is happening beneath one's touch. It is important to have good instruction in skeletal and myofascial anatomy, as well as recognition of the placement and function of internal organs. It is also helpful to learn about the layers of skin and the superficial fascia (adipose layer), as they contain a richness of blood vessels, nerve endings, and glands. Therapists who are knowledgeable in anatomy convey a sense of competence and inspire confidence in the people they touch.[1-4]

Awareness of Breath and Grounding

It is important to maintain an awareness of your breath as you practice Comfort Touch. Your breathing should be easy and natural throughout the session. The effectiveness of the techniques is enhanced by the conscious use of your breath. When holding a general area or a specific point longer than the usual 1½ seconds used when following a sequence, coordinate the hold with your breath. The pressure might then be held throughout the cycle of one or two of your respirations.

During a session, it is *not* necessary to request that the client breathe deliberately. For example, saying to the client, "Take a deep breath" can actually be counterproductive, as it interferes with the client's relaxation. It can be confusing, or feel like an imposition to the client. The experienced therapist will notice that by breathing fully and deeply oneself, the client will naturally follow.

At all times maintain your sense of grounding, the feeling of connection to the earth. Be aware of the placement of your feet. As you apply pressure with your hands on the client, also be aware of, and/or apply pressure downward with the soles of your feet.

By doing so, you maintain coherence throughout your nervous system, which greatly enhances the effectiveness of your work. The client also will feel your touch more deeply, and benefit by the feeling of your connection to the earth.

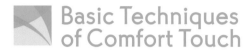

Basic Techniques of Comfort Touch

The following techniques can all be practiced by applying varying degrees of pressure on the client. It should feel firm, but never forced, "pokey," or too deep. For general or broad contact, begin with 2 pounds of pressure, gradually increasing the pressure up to 4 or 5 pounds, depending on the condition and preferences of the client. When working on large areas of the body, such as the arms, legs, or back, determine the general level of pressure appropriate to the person, and apply that pressure consistently to the area. For example, for a frail, elderly client, you might apply pressure in the range or 2–4 pounds. For a younger person, or one with more muscle tone, you might apply pressure closer to the range of 5–7 pounds. The client's feedback will be your guide throughout the session.

For more specific strokes the pressure may be only 1 to 3 pounds, causing only slight indentation to the skin. You can use a small, flat kitchen scale that measures in pounds and ounces to get a sense of the appropriate amount of pressure, as illustrated in Figure 5-1. The broader the contact, the greater the amount of pressure that can be exerted.

When beginning to use any of these techniques with clients, ask for their feedback on the amount of pressure, and monitor their verbal and nonverbal feedback throughout. In working with young, healthy indi-

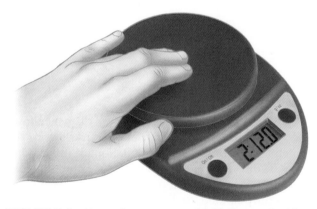

FIGURE 5-1. Measuring pressure with kitchen scale. Use of a kitchen scale can help you learn to gauge your pressure in applying Comfort Touch techniques. The broader the contact, the greater the amount of pressure that can be exerted.

viduals you may use more pressure, according to the client's needs and preferences. It is important that your pressure be consistent. As the client becomes familiar with your touch, she or he can relax. Consistency of contact throughout a session contributes to the experience of comfort and safety for the client.

Following the description of each technique there will be an example of how it is used and applied in a Comfort Touch session.

Encompassing

This technique is especially suitable for the limbs. Hold the body part (arm, hand, leg, or foot) between your hands. Let your thumbs be parallel to each other, to avoid poking pressure with the tips of the thumbs. As you begin with this technique, you can picture your hands with the thumbs parallel so that the fingers spread out to form the image of a butterfly as in Figure 5-2.

The "wings" of the butterfly wrap around the part of the body you are touching. Use the full surfaces of your hands to contact and encompass that body part. Pressure is firm and evenly distributed as shown in Figure 5-3. It is important that the palms of your hands contact the client's body. Your thumb tips and fingertips will be relaxed, not poking into the client.

Example: The client may be either seated in a chair or lying in a bed. To work on the arm, begin by encompassing the upper arm, gently pressing into the center of the arm with both hands as in Figure 5-3. Continue to move down the length of the arm, releasing pressure between each placement of your hands. Maintain

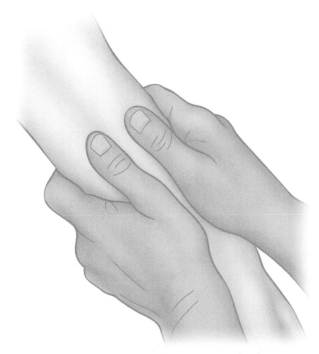

FIGURE 5-3. Encompassing the arm. Use the full surfaces of your hands to contact and encompass the arm with firm, even pressure.

a steady and easy rhythm of contact as you sequence down the arm. Each placement of your hands lasts about 1½ to 2 seconds. Encompass the whole surface of the hand, including the thumb and fingers.

Broad Contact Pressure

This technique is used to apply compression to one area of the body or series of points. It is appropriate for the large areas of the back, parallel and lateral to the spine. Pressure can be applied with the whole hand, the palm or heel of the hand, or the base of the thumb. The amount of force exerted ranges from 3 to 6 pounds of pressure. For this technique the client may be seated in a regular chair or a wheelchair. Another option is to have the client sit on the edge of the bed, as you sit beside her or him to apply contact pressure.

Example: With the client seated in a regular chair or wheelchair, stand at her or his left side with your left hand gently holding the left shoulder. Place the heel of your right hand at the top of the erector spinae muscles to the right of the spinal column, as shown in Figure 5-4.

Press into the body, at a 90° angle to the surface of the skin. Hold the pressure for 2 to 3 seconds. Release, and continue to move down the length of the erector spinae muscles, through the mid-back as shown in

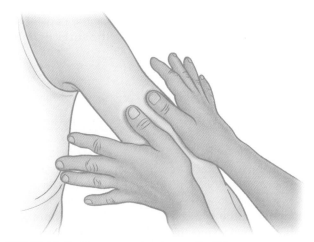

FIGURE 5-2. Encompassing butterfly. When encompassing the arm or leg, let your thumbs be parallel, letting your outstretched fingers form the shape of a butterfly. The "wings" of the butterfly wrap around the part of the body you are touching.

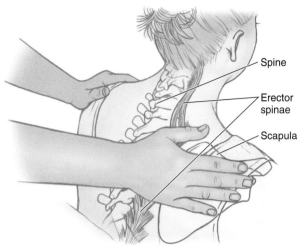

FIGURE 5-4. Broad contact pressure on upper back. Apply pressure with the heel of the hand into the erector spinae muscles which are lateral to the spine and medial to the scapula. Press into the body, at a 90° angle, and hold for 2–3 seconds.

Figure 5-5, pressing with each placement of the heel of your hand.

Let the client move forward slightly, as you continue to support her or him with your left hand, and apply pressure to the erectors muscles of the lower back with the right hand. The back of your forearm is contacting and pressing against the back of the chair to gain leverage as necessary. Move down until you reach the base of the back. Apply pressure directly to the sacrum with the surfaces of your fingers as shown in Figure 5-6. (You may sit on a stool beside the client to work on the low back and sacrum.) This pressure on the sacrum tends to be very calming for the client.

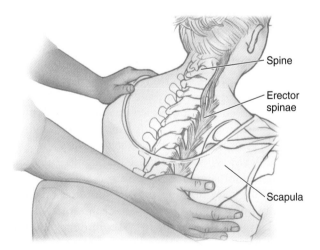

FIGURE 5-5. Broad contact pressure on mid-back. Apply broad contact pressure with your right hand to the right side of the client's back. As you continue to press down the client's back, keep your arm in contact with the back of the chair, using it for leverage.

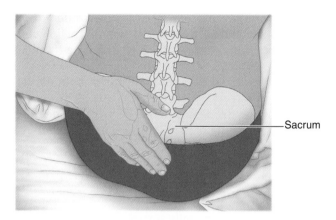

FIGURE 5-6. Broad contact pressure on sacrum. Apply pressure directly over the sacrum, and hold for few seconds. This is very calming for the client.

Move to the other side and repeat the sequence while standing to her or his right, with your right hand on the client's right shoulder. Apply pressure to the erector spinae muscles of the left side of the back. End with contact pressure on the sacrum.

Specific Contact Pressure

Specific contact pressure is used to contact a smaller or more specific area than with *broad contact pressure.* Usually you would use broad contact pressure to warm the area before applying more specific pressure. If a person is very sensitive or ticklish (eg, on the soles of the feet), avoid specific contact pressure and stay with the broad contact.

Examples: Use the broad flat surfaces of the fingertips to apply specific contact pressure to the palm and heel of the hand (see Figure 5-7). Use the pads of the thumbs (not the tips) to press into the surfaces of the foot (see Figure 5-8).

Broad Contact Circling

This technique is always used in combination with *broad contact pressure.* The intention is to get deeper into the layers of bodies tissues, e.g., the fascia and the muscle. First, contact pressure is applied. Maintaining pressure and contact, rotate one-and-a-quarter turns, as if *spiraling* to a deeper layer (see Figure 5-9). The diameter of the spiral is very small, only about ¼ to ½ inch. When using the right hand, the direction of rotation is clockwise; when using the left hand the direction of rotation is counterclockwise. Remember that the circling does *not* happen at the surface of the skin, creating friction on the skin. Use this technique only when you feel the tissue of the client *allowing* this

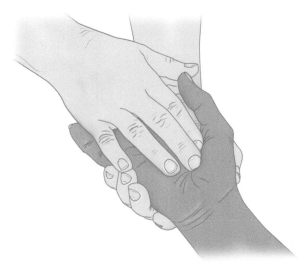

FIGURE 5-7. **Specific contact pressure on the hand.** While holding the client's hand with one of your hands, use the flat surfaces of the fingertips of your other hand to press into the palm and the heel of the hand.

entry into the tissue below the surface. Never push your way deeper.

Use broad contact circling in areas of greater density in the body, e.g., into the belly of the erector spinae muscles of the back, large muscles of the upper arm (deltoid, biceps femoris), or upper leg (quadriceps).

Example: Use broad contact circling on the deltoid muscle. Begin by encompassing the shoulder joint. Let one hand slide on top of the shoulder, as the other

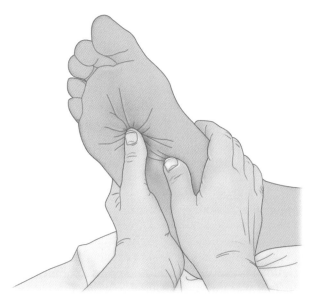

FIGURE 5-8. **Specific contact pressure on the foot.** While encompassing the foot with both hands, use the pads of the thumbs (not the tips) to press into the surfaces of the foot.

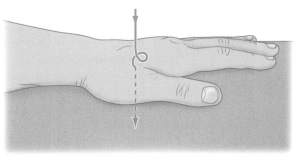

FIGURE 5-9. **Broad contact circling.** Begin by touching the body with broad contact pressure. Maintaining pressure and contact, rotate one-and-a-quarter turn, as if spiraling into a deeper layer. Continue to press directly into center for a few seconds. (The long arrow represents the direction of pressure and the small spiral represents the movement of the hand as it goes deeper into the body.)

hand presses into the deltoid muscle on the outside of the shoulder. Maintaining pressure and contact, rotate one-and-a-quarter turns, as if *spiraling* in to a deeper layer of the body as shown in Figure 5-10.

Specific Contact Circling

This technique is used in combination with *specific contact pressure.* The intention is to get deeper into a specific area, where a smaller area of contact is most effective at relieving tension. First, specific contact pressure is

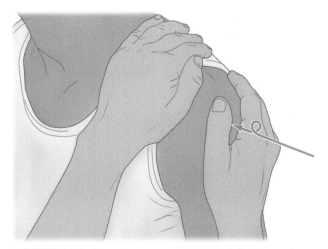

FIGURE 5-10. **Broad contact circling on deltoid muscle.** The left hand encompasses the shoulder while the right hand applies contact pressure to the deltoid muscle. Maintaining pressure and contact, rotate one-and-a-quarter turns clockwise with the right hand, as if spiraling in to a deeper layer. (The long arrow represents the direction of pressure and the small spiral represents the movement of the hand as it goes deeper into the body.)

applied. Maintaining pressure and contact, rotate one-and-a-quarter turns, as if *spiraling* into a deeper layer. The diameter of the spiral is very small, no more than ¼ inch. When using the right hand, the direction of rotation is clockwise; when using the left hand the direction of rotation is counterclockwise. The circling does *not* happen at the surface of the skin, creating friction. Use this technique only when you feel the tissue of the client *allowing* this entry into the tissue below the surface. Never push your way deeper.

Specific contact pressure is usually applied to areas of greatest muscular tension (e.g., the belly of the trapezius muscle); or to areas of greater tissue density (e.g., the calluses around the heels of the feet). It is also used with specific therapeutic acupressure points (e.g., the belly of the brachioradialis muscle).

Example: Use specific contact circling into the motor point of the trapezius muscle. As the left hand provides broad encompassing contact on the left shoulder, the middle finger of the right hand presses into the motor point of the right side of the trapezius muscle. Maintaining pressure and contact, rotate one-and-a-quarter turns, as if spiraling into a deeper layer of the muscle as shown in Figure 5-11.

The motor point in the belly of the trapezius muscle is also called Gallbladder 21 or "shoulder well" in traditional acupressure. Usually it is best to apply broad contact pressure to warm this area before applying specific contact pressure or specific contact circling. See Figures 4-6 and Figure 5-12. Whether using broad or

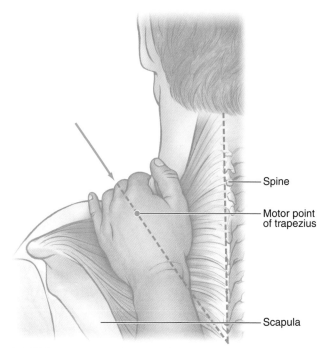

FIGURE 5-12. "Shoulder Well." Apply broad contact pressure to the belly of the trapezius muscle, before applying specific contact pressure and contact circling.

specific pressure to this point, remember that it is applied perpendicularly to the surface of the skin, and is directed into the central axis of the body. Even 2–3 minutes of well-placed pressure to this point can have tremendous benefit in alleviating pain and tension in the neck and shoulders.

Additional Techniques of Comfort Touch

While the basic techniques of Comfort Touch are the ones most frequently used, there are additional techniques that have merit for particular effects.

Encompassing Lift and Squeeze

Encompassing lift and squeeze is used to take hold of a specific muscle and squeeze into the mass of the muscle itself. It is used in limited areas of greater muscular tension only in clients with higher levels of muscle tone (not where there is fragile skin or blood vessels). This technique is especially useful to relieve shoulder tension. It is also appropriate in other larger muscle areas that can easily be isolated (eg, the brachioradialis muscle of the lower arm and the gastrocnemius muscle of the lower leg).

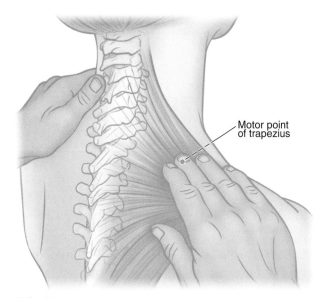

FIGURE 5-11. Specific contact circling into the motor point of the trapezius muscle: The middle finger of the right hand presses into the motor point of the trapezius muscle. Maintaining pressure and contact, rotate one-and-a-quarter turns, as if spiraling into a deeper layer of the muscle.

Hints for Practice

SCRIBE

Before beginning a session of Comfort Touch, silently recite the principles of Comfort Touch—SCRIBE—to yourself. Many practitioners have found this a useful practice: As you think of the first principle—slow—take a moment to breathe fully, and feel yourself deeply grounded and connected to the earth. With the thoughts of comforting and respectful, you set your intention and attitude to be with the client in the present circumstance. As you think of into center, broad, and encompassing, you are reminding yourself of the techniques you will use.

Even during the session, you can repeat these six words silently to yourself, particularly if you are feeling uncertain about what to do at any point. Repetition of the words will clarify your intention and bring focus to your application of the techniques, increasing your confidence and enjoyment in providing the gift of touch to others.

Example: With the client in the seated position, lift the bellies of the trapezius muscle with the broad surfaces the hands—not the fingertips. Squeeze into the mass of the muscle, and release (see Figure 5-13). This is an area of significant muscular tension for many people, regardless of age or level of physical activity. This broad squeezing pressure allows a release of the constriction in the fascia surrounding the muscle fibers, in turn freeing the constriction of nerves, and allowing greater flow of nutrients through the blood vessels.

Lifting and squeezing the belly of the middle trapezius muscle, as shown, effectively accesses the motor points of the muscle. It can be held for 2–7 seconds, depending on the feedback of the client. Some clients may want to slowly move their heads on their own as you hold pressure to this point. In this way they can gently stretch the muscles of the neck. This is a very useful technique to use for medical staff and other caregivers in settings where Comfort Touch is practiced.

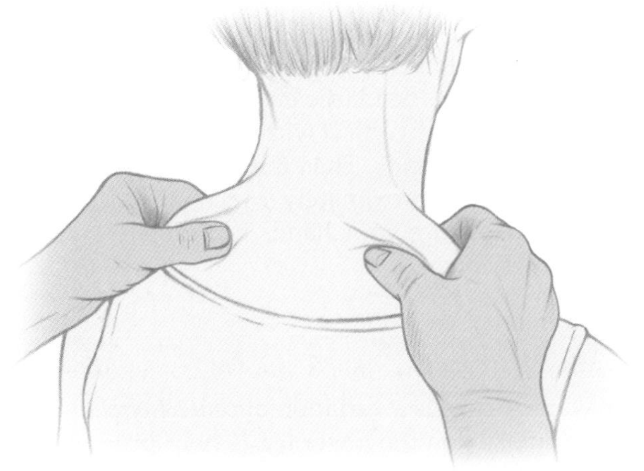

Encompassing Joint or Limb Movement

In this technique, the intention is to introduce a gentle movement to the part of the body being touched. Not only is this helpful in increasing local circulation of blood and lymph, but it contributes to a feeling of freedom and ease for the client. It is usually performed in combination with *encompassing* or *contact pressure.* As the body part is touched, lift it and very gently move it in space in a slow circular or wavelike motion. Unlike typical range-of-motion exercises, the intention here is *not* to test or extend the range of motion. Nor is the intention to stretch a limb or pull on a joint. The technique can be used when encompassing the shoulder joint, the arm, or hand. It can also be used when encompassing the feet.

Example: Place the broad surfaces of your hands around the shoulder joint, encompassing the whole joint. Gently lifting the shoulder, move it in a very small circular motion (see Figure 5-14).

Example: While encompassing the hand, introduce a gentle circular or wavelike motion to the hand and forearm. With one hand supporting the elbow of the client, you can lift the whole arm gently and move it, being careful not to stretch or strain the client's shoulder joint.

Broad Contact Brushing

This technique is used as a finishing stroke after using other techniques on a particular part of the body, such as the arm or leg. Using the full palmar surface of one

FIGURE 5-13. Lift and squeeze trapezius muscle. Lift the bellies of the trapezius muscle with the broad, surfaces of the thumbs and the fingers—not the fingertips. Squeeze into the mass of the muscle, and release.

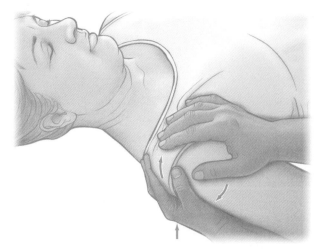

FIGURE 5-14. Encompassing joint movement of the shoulder. While <u>encompassing</u> the shoulder joint, incorporate movement by gently lifting the shoulder and moving it in a small

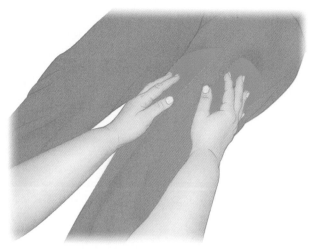

FIGURE 5-15. Broad contact brushing on the legs. Using the palmar surfaces of your hands, contact and brush down the client's leg.

or both hands, let your hand trace down the length of the body part being touched. This conveys a soothing sense of release. The contact should be firm enough not to be ticklish or too stimulating, but not so firm as to be uncomfortable or damaging (8–16 ounces of pressure). It is a stroke that acknowledges the flow of energy down the body, reinforcing a sense of relaxation. Do not use this stroke if the person is ticklish, or particularly sensitive, or does not respond well to it.

In the seated position, broad contact brushing can be used to brush from the top of the head, down the sides of the head, onto the shoulders. It is also used to brush down the arms. In the supine position it is used after working on the shoulders, arms, and hands, brushing down the length of the limb to finish. Likewise, you can brush down the length of the legs and feet after working on them. The stroke is done relatively quickly (about 3 seconds to cover the length of the arm), but not too fast. Brushing is often followed by holding a specific point to end the session. For example, after brushing the legs, the feet may be held for a few seconds.

Example. With the client in the supine position, use broad contact brushing after having completed work on the legs. Using the palmar surfaces of your hands, let your hands contact and trace down the client's leg. Hold the feet for a few seconds to finish work on the leg (see Figure 5-15).

Holding—Contact and Non-contact

Holding is most often used to begin or end a sequence of touch on a particular part of the body. To begin a session, it establishes the connection between the therapist and client, giving the client a chance to experience the warm and calming influence of the contact. When hold-

ing, let your contact be firm and encompassing, with the contact lasting approximately 5 seconds. Holding may be applied to any body part, such as the hands, the feet, or the head.

Holding also provides a useful and satisfying way to close a session; for example, when applied to the abdominal or sternal regions. When holding as a closing stroke, hold for a few seconds, then release your contact and move your hands away from the client's body 1 to 2 inches. Hold your hands in a position of *non-contact holding* for a few seconds, then release your hands, letting them come completely away from the client's body. This allows a clear and precise transition that conveys that you are finished with the sequence, but you are not rushing away from the person.

Example: Use holding and non-contact holding to close a session with a client who is in the supine position. Standing at the client's right side, place your right hand on the abdomen and place your left hand at the top of the person's head (see Figure 5-16).

Both hands will contact with 1 to 2 pounds of pressure for 3 to 7 seconds. Then move your hands away from the body approximately 1 inch, and hold for a few seconds. Bring your hands completely away to close the session.

Water Stroke

The water stroke is a variation of *contact circling*. It is used primarily on the lower leg to help promote circulation of lymph, and provide relief from edema or swelling of the lower leg and ankles. To perform the water stroke place the fingertips of all fingers on the area being touched. Exerting only about 6 to 8 *ounces* of pressure, contact the skin and make very small cir-

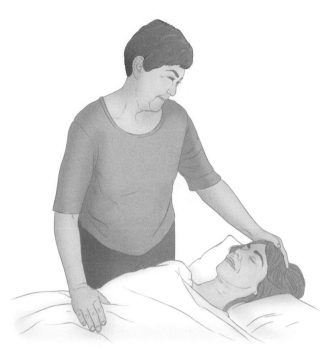

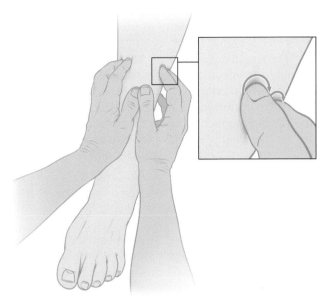

FIGURE 5-16. Contact and noncontact holding to end a session. Place your right hand over the abdomen and your left hand at the top of the client's head. Hold 1–2 pounds of pressure for 3–7 seconds. Move your hands away from the body approximately 1 inch and hold for a few seconds, before bringing your hands completely away to close the session.

FIGURE 5-17. Water stroke on the lower leg. Fingertips (not thumbs) are placed on either side of the tibia bone, midway down the legs. Exerting 6–8 <u>ounces</u> of pressure, make very small circles with the fingertips of each hand. Move the fingertips one-half inch lower and repeat. Continue down the leg and onto the top of the foot and the sides of the heel.

cles in one place; move about half an inch away and repeat the movement. When done correctly, it is very relaxing for the patient. Imagine as you perform this stroke that the fluid in the subcutaneous layer of the body is slowly moving toward the heart. (Note: In many cases edema is relieved by use of this stroke, but in cases of extreme swelling—for example, in advanced heart disease and cancer—it will not be effective and *any* touch to the area may be painful. Avoid touch if it causes pain to the patient.)

Example: Sit at the patient's feet and place the fingertips of both hands midway down one of the lower legs of the patient. Fingertips should be placed on either side of the tibia bone, resting in a natural placement on the patient's body (see Figure 5-17). Contact and make very small circles with the fingertips of each hand. Move the fingertips ½ inch lower and repeat. Continue all the way down the leg and on to the top of the foot and the sides of the heel. Repeat the sequence on the other leg.

Moisturizing the Skin

Because the techniques of Comfort Touch *do not rub* the skin or otherwise create friction on the tissues, they do not require the application of lotion of oils.

Furthermore, it is recommended for the beginning practitioner *not* to use lubricants, in order to avoid the habit of relying on them and reverting to the use of gliding or kneading strokes of conventional massage. However, there are times when the use of an unscented moisturizing lotion is indicated, and it may be applied with a slow, broad encompassing stroke sufficient to moisturize the skin. Lotion may be applied to the dry skin when it is appropriate, with the permission of the client or the client's caregiver. Sometimes lotion is used at the individual's request for its soothing, sensual appeal.

Example: Apply lotion to the feet or hands with slow, broad, encompassing pressure. It can be especially useful if the skin is very dry or itchy. Use only a high-quality unscented lotion, or use something that is already familiar to the client to avoid allergic or hypersensitive reactions.

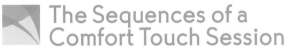

The Sequences of a Comfort Touch Session

Comfort Touch is performed on clients in the position that is most comfortable, safe, and appropriate for them. The following are three of the most common positions used in this work, with suggested sequences for each: the seated position, the supine position, and the side-lying position. In practice there is room for variations on these, owing to the specific needs and preferences of the client.

The length of a session may vary from 10 to 20 minutes, if focusing on one area of the body, to as much as 50 minutes, if working on the whole body. Never spend more than 60 minutes of hands-on time with clients, as this can be too much input for them and actually can be tiring. The average length of time for a Comfort Touch session in many hospices, hospitals, and homecare settings is 30–40 minutes.

Seated Position

For this sequence the client may be seated in a regular chair or a wheelchair. (For someone who is seated in a recliner, follow the sequence outlined below in the Supine Position.) Use a towel or small pillow, if necessary, to help support the back in proper alignment, and to pad the back of the chair. The seated position is useful for the client because it helps to encourage good posture and facilitates easy, full breathing. It is also easy to access most of the body.

Shoulders, Back, Arms, and Hands

1. **Top of shoulder:** Standing behind the client, place your hands at the top of the client's shoulders using *contact pressure.* The palms of the hands are placed directly on the bellies of the client's trapezius muscles (the thickest part of the muscle straight down from the ears). Take time to feel the breath of the client through the palms of your hands. Pressure is then applied perpendicularly (at a 90° angle) to the surface of the client's skin and directed into the central axis of the client's body.

2. **Trapezius motor point:** Use *specific contact pressure* to the belly (motor point) of the trapezius muscle, doing one side at a time. Use *contact circling* with the heel of the hand or pads of the fingers to the belly of the trapezius muscle, doing one side at a time (see Figures 5-11 and 5-12).

3. **Upper back:** Standing at the client's left side, use the heel of your right hand to apply *contact pressure* to the erector spinae muscles on the right side of the body. The erector muscles are lateral to the spine and medial to the scapula. Pressure is directed *in* to the mass of the muscles. Do not push the muscles in any direction, simply press *into* them. The other hand is on the left shoulder to provide gentle support and stability (see Figure 5-4).

4. **Mid and lower back:** Continue down the erector muscles on the right side of the client's back with *contact pressure.* Press each placement of the hand for approximately 1½ to 2 seconds. Continue all the way down the erectors using *contact pressure.* As you get below the level of the back of the chair, use the padded (with towel) back of the chair for leverage. Continue to stand (or sit on a stool) at the person's left side, allowing your arm and hand to be between the person and the chair back (see Figure 5-5).

5. **Sacrum:** When you get to the base of the spine, place the palm of your hand directly on the client's sacrum and apply *contact pressure* (see Figure 5-6).

6. **Repeat steps 3, 4, and 5 on the left side of the back.** You will be using your left hand to apply *contact pressure,* and your right hand will rest on the client's right shoulder to provide gentle support.

7. **Shoulder joint:** You may sit on a stool or chair beside the client. With both hands *encompass* the shoulder joint. Let the warmth of your hands penetrate into the shoulder. You may apply *encompassing joint movement* to the whole joint as you *encompass* it (see Figure 5-14).

8. **Upper arm:** *Encompass* the upper arm. Notice that the shape of your hands forms a *butterfly* (see Figure 5-2). The thumbs are parallel to each other with the fingers opened out to the side. Pressure is applied evenly all around the arm. It is especially important that the palms of your hands make firm contact, while the rest of the hand simply wraps around the arm. (Do not poke or press in with the thumbs or fingertips, as this can cause discomfort and/or bruising or tearing of the skin.) Move down the arm, holding each placement of the hands for approximately 1½ seconds (see Figure 5-3).

9. **Lower arm:** *Encompass* the elbow. *Encompass* the lower arm. One hand is held on top of the arm; the other hand is held beneath the arm. Maintain even pressure all around the arm. Move down the arm, holding each placement of your hands for approximately 1½ seconds.

10. **Hand:** *Encompass* the hand, also using general and specific *contact pressure* on all the surfaces of the hand (see Figure 5-7). Apply pressure to the thumbs and fingers, *encompassing* both the top and bottom and sides of each digit. Use *broad contact brushing* to smooth down the length of the arm from shoulder to fingertips.

11. **Repeat Steps 7 through 10 for the other shoulder, arm, and hand.**

Hips, Legs, and Feet

1. **Hip and upper leg:** Use *broad contact pressure* on the hip and upper leg. The hands give broad pressure *into* the central axis of the leg. (If the client is in a wheelchair, you can remove the arms from the chair for better access.) With one hand use *encompassing broad contact pressure* on the outside of the leg. The other hand is placed on top of the thigh, also using *encompassing broad contact pressure.* Move downward and diagonally across the top of the thigh with each placement of the hands, eventually reaching the inside of the knee. In other words, the medial hand is perpendicular to and follows the pathway of the sartorius muscle in its placements. Fingertips are pointing toward the hip joints. See Figure 5-18.
2. **Knee:** *Encompass* the knee. One hand is on the knee, while the other hand is behind it and supporting the joint. Let the warmth from your hands penetrate the joint.
3. **Lower leg:** Use *broad contact pressure* and/or *encompassing* down the leg. Move down the leg, holding each placement of the hands for approximately 1½ seconds.
4. **Feet:** Use *broad contact pressure* and *encompassing* on all the surfaces of the foot. Change your body position to get comfortable as you work. You may sit on a chair or small stool.
5. **Repeat Steps 1 through 4 on the other side.**

Head and Closing

1. **Head:** *Encompass* the head. Place your hand at the back of the neck, with full hand contact. The other hand gently supports the forehead. The intention here is to allow the weight of the person's head to rest between your hands.
   a. **Occipital ridge:** Use *specific contact pressure* and *specific contact circling* along the occipital ridge at the base of the skull—*not* into the neck itself. See Figure 5-19.
   (Important note: Do **not** use specific pressure into the neck itself. The structures of the neck with its bony protuberances, including the spinous and transverse processes of the cervical vertebrae, along with the major blood vessels, including the carotid and vertebral arteries, are generally too vulnerable to work into safely. The *contact circling* of the occipital ridge and *specific contact pressure* in the belly of the trapezius muscle are usually very effective in alleviating neck pain, without the potential for injury posed by working specifically on the neck itself.)
   b. **Scalp:** Stand behind the client and place your hands on either side of the head. Hold the head in your hands gently while taking a deep full breath. Allow the client

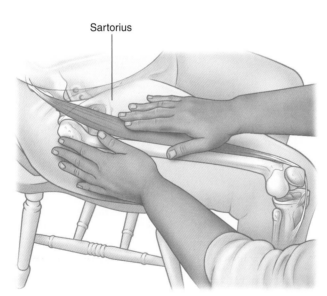

FIGURE 5-18. Hip and upper leg. With the left hand on the outside of the leg, and the right hand on the top of the thigh, use broad contact pressure into the central axis of the leg. The right hand is perpendicular to and follows the pathway of the sartorius muscle, as the left hand remains on the outside of the leg.

Sartorius

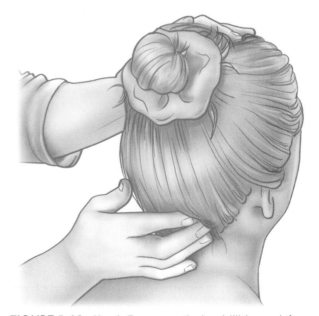

FIGURE 5-19. Head. Encompass the head. With your left hand gently supporting the head, use the fingers and/or thumb of your right hand to do specific contact pressure and specific contact circling along the occipital ridge at the base of the skull. Be sure the pressure is on the occipital ridge—not into the neck itself.

to feel the support of your hands, as well as the expansiveness that comes with the cycle of the breath. Use gentle *contact circling* on the scalp.

2. **Closing:** Use *broad contact brushing* to smooth the hair. Place the hands on the shoulders and *hold* through a full breath. Bring your hands an inch away from the body and *hold* for a few seconds. Release your hands down to your side to end the session.

Supine Position

The client can be in a bed, with or without a head lift. Pillows are used to support the neck and spine in proper alignment, and to allow for the comfort of the client. A soft feather or down pillow usually gives the greatest comfort to the neck. Pillows are placed under the knees for support, allowing for relaxation of the low back muscles. If using a hospital bed, you can adjust the height of the bed to a comfortable level to work. If using a regular bed or massage table that is lower, you can sit comfortably on a stool for most of the treatment, if you prefer.

This sequence is also used for a client who is seated in a recliner. The recliner gives opportunities for a number of different levels of incline, so let the client determine what is most comfortable for her or him. Use pillows or small towels if necessary, to enhance her or his comfort. For some of the steps in the sequence below, you may need to make minor adjustments, due to the wings of the back of the recliner. Remember that your comfort as a practitioner is also very important to the success of a session, so avoid doing anything which is difficult or uncomfortable to either you or your client.

Neck, Shoulders, Arms, and Hands

1. **C-7 hold:** Begin at the client's right side. With the client in the supine position, place your left hand under the base of the neck, supporting the area around the 7th cervical vertebrae (C-7). The hand is relaxed and cupped to encompass the joint. Do *not* put pressure on the vertebra itself. The right hand is placed on top of the shoulder to *encompass* the shoulder region. Hold for 5 to 10 seconds. See Figure 5-20.

2. **Trapezius motor point:** With your right hand continuing to *encompass* on the front of the shoulder joint (anterior deltoid muscle), the left hand moves into position to palpate the belly of the trapezius muscle. *Lift and squeeze* this muscle. Use *contact pressure* into the motor point (also called gallbladder-21 or "shoulder well" in traditional acupressure) within the

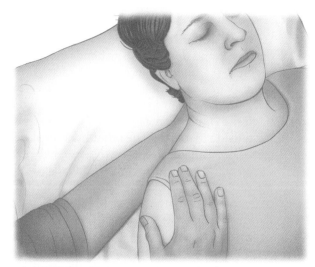

FIGURE 5-20. C-7 hold. With the right hand placed lightly on top of the shoulder, place the left hand under the client's neck, supporting the area around the 7th cervical vertebrae (C-7). The hand is relaxed and cupped to avoid placing pressure on the vertebrae itself.

belly of this muscle. Use *specific contact circling* into this point. See Figure 5-21.

3. **Shoulder:** With the left hand underneath the shoulder and the right hand on top, *encompass* the shoulder with both hands, allowing the warmth of your hands to penetrate into the joint. You may apply *encompassing joint movement* to the whole joint as you *encompass* it (see Figure 5-14).

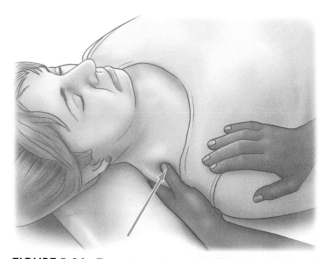

FIGURE 5-21. Trapezius motor point. With your right hand resting lightly on the front of the shoulder, the left hand lifts and squeezes the belly of the trapezius muscle. Use contact pressure and specific contact circling into the motor point of the muscle.

4. **Arm:** Use *encompassing contact pressure* down the length of the arm. For the upper arm, keep the hands in the position of the *butterfly press* (see Figure 5-2) with the thumbs parallel, and fingers wrapping outward around the arm (see Figure 5-3). *Encompass* the elbow. *Encompass* the lower arm. One of your hands is held on top, the other hand held beneath the arm. Maintain even pressure all around the arm. Move down the arm, holding each placement of your hands for approximately 1½ seconds.

5. **Hand:** Use *encompassing contact pressure,* holding the client's hand between your hands. While holding the client's hand (dorsal side up) with your left hand, use the flat part of the fingertips and thumb of your right hand to exert *encompassing pressure* into the length of the thumb and each finger. With the client's hand palmar side up, use *general* and *specific contact pressure* on the surface of the palm (see Figure 5-7).

6. **Tonic acupressure points:** Holding the client's wrist with your left hand, hold the client's hand in your right hand (as if to shake it), press with the pad of your right thumb into the web of the client's thumb and index finger (see Figure 5-22). Hold for a few seconds. Continue holding the client's hand with your right hand as you encompass the lower arm just below the elbow with your left hand. Let the pad of the thumb of your left hand sink into the belly of the brachioradialis muscle (see Figure 5-23). Hold for a few seconds.

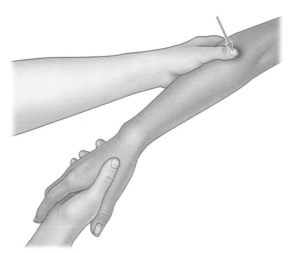

FIGURE 5-23. Tonic point in forearm: While gently holding the client's right hand, press with the pad of your left thumb into the belly of the brachioradialis muscle. Hold for a few seconds.

7. **Brush arm:** Use *broad contact brushing* to smooth down the length of the arm from shoulder to fingertips.

8. **Repeat Steps 1 through 7 on the client's left side.**

Hips, Legs, and Feet

1. **Hip and upper leg:** Use *broad encompassing contact pressure* over the hip and upper leg. Your hands give broad pressure into the central axis of the leg. With one hand use *broad contact pressure* on the outside of the leg. The other hand is placed on top of the thigh, moving downward and diagonally across the top of the thigh with each placement of the hands, eventually reaching the inside of the knee. In other words, the medial hand is parallel to and follows the pathway of the sartorius muscle in its placements. Fingertips are pointing toward the hip joints. See Figure 5-24.

2. **Knee:** Lift the knee to *encompass* it. One hand is on top of the knee with the other hand behind and supporting the joint. Let the warmth from the hands penetrate the joint.

3. **Lower leg:** Use *broad contact pressure* and/or *encompassing* down the leg. Move down the leg, holding each placement of the hands for approximately 1½ seconds.

4. **Foot:** Use *encompassing contact pressure* on the entire surface of the foot. Use *specific contact pressure* and *contact circling* to thoroughly massage the bottom of the foot. Do not use the tips

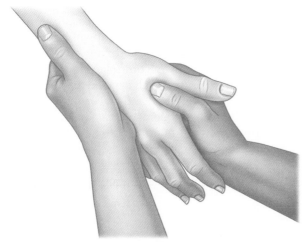

FIGURE 5-22. Tonic point in hand. While holding the client's wrist with your left hand, press into the web of the client's thumb and index finger with your pad of your right thumb. Hold for a few seconds.

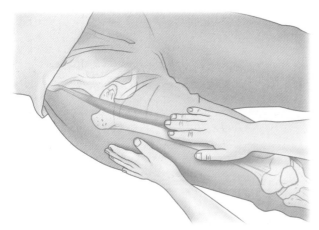

FIGURE 5-24. Hip and upper leg: With your left hand on the outside of the client's leg, and your right hand on top of the client's leg, give broad encompassing contact pressure to the hip and upper leg. With each placement of the hands, the right hand follows the pathway of the sartorius muscle. Keep the fingertips pointing toward the hip joints.

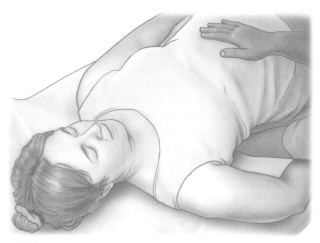

FIGURE 5-25. Abdomen and low back. Place your left hand under the small of the client's low back, and rest your right hand lightly on the abdomen. Feel the weight of the client's back sink downward as you encompass the low back and belly. Keeping your top hand in contact with the client's belly, let it rise and sink as it follows the movement of the

of your fingers; rather, use the broader surfaces of the pads of your fingers and thumbs (see Figure 5-8). While most of this work is done through the person's clothing, you may remove the client's sock to work on the foot. If the sock is removed, put it back on after working on the foot.

5. **Repeat Steps 1 through 4 on the client's other side.**

Abdomen, Low Back, Upper Torso, and Head

1. **Abdomen and low back:** Stand or sit at the client's right side. Place your left hand under the small of the client's low back. Place the right hand lightly on the abdomen. Allow the weight of the client's back to sink down into your left hand. With the upper hand resting gently on the belly, *encompass* the low back and the belly, paying particular attention to the client's breath (see Figure 5-25). Let your hand follow the movement of the client's breath, rising and sinking several times with the breath. (Note: It is *not* necessary to ask the client to "take a breath" or to direct the breath in any way. If the therapist is breathing fully and deeply, the client will inevitably follow.) This encompassing hold allows for relaxation of the muscles of the low back and the abdomen.

2. **Upper torso:** Place your left hand under the back of the client's neck. Place the fingertips of

your right hand lightly on the client's upper chest over the mid-sternum. *Encompass* and *hold* the upper torso, paying attention to the client's breath, allowing her or him to expand the chest with each inhalation (see Figure 5-26).

3. **Head:** While your left hand remains under the client's neck, place the palm of your right hand on the client's forehead, exerting *light contact pressure.* (If it is not comfortable for either you or the client to have your left hand under the head, you can, instead, rest your left hand lightly on the client's right shoulder.) Use the flat surfaces of your fingertips to do *contact circling* on the forehead between the eyebrows. Use light contact pressure along the brow line. With the fingertips of both hands, you can do *light contact circling* on both of the temples at the same time (see Figure 5-27).

4. **Closing:** Place your left hand on the client's forehead or top of head, and place your right hand on the client's abdomen. *Hold* for a few seconds (see Figure 5-16). Bring both hands away from the body an inch or two. Use *noncontact holding* for a few seconds. Then bring your hands down to your side to end the sequence.

Side-Lying Position

The side-lying position is a very comfortable position for many people, and it allows easy access to apply the techniques of Comfort Touch to the back. Other

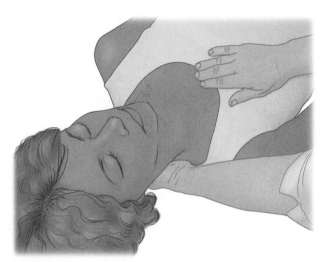

FIGURE 5-26. Upper torso: Your left hand gently supports the back of the client's neck, while the fingertips of your right hand contact the sternum. <u>Encompass</u> and <u>hold,</u> keeping your pressure light enough to allow the client to expand his or her chest with each inhalation.

parts of the body can be contacted in this position as well, though it is primarily used to work on the back. To work in the side-lying position, begin by allowing clients to roll onto the side that is most comfortable to them. (When the client has limited mobility, it is typical to work with the person only on one side.) Place a pillow underneath the head, so that it is in proper alignment with the spine. Place a pillow between the legs and knees. The client may also enjoy leaning on or hugging a pillow placed in front of her or his torso.

1. **Shoulder:** *Encompass* the shoulder that is on top. Use *contact pressure* and *lift and squeeze* in the bellies of the trapezius muscles.
2. **Back.** Use *contact pressure* on the back, along the erector spinae muscles, lateral to the spine. Work first along one side of the spine, and then on the other. Keep your pressure broad, consistent, and firm. *Never* press on the spine itself. If the client is lying on her or his right side, your left hand will be parallel to the spine, pressing the erector spinae muscles. Always keep the angle of your wrist neutral (not at a sharp angle) to avoid stressing your wrist joint. Your right hand can be used to apply direct pressure to the back of your left hand, giving it added support (see Figure 5-28). As you move down the back, hold each placement of the hands for approximately 1½ to 2 seconds.

    Contact pressure can also applied with the back of your hand, using the fist of the other hand to give strength and stability to the press. Let the back of the hand that is in contact with the client's body be soft. If done correctly, the client will find it difficult to tell what surface of your hand is touching her or him (see Figure 5-29).
3. **The sacrum:** Use *contact pressure* directly on the sacrum. Hold *contact pressure* on the sacrum and the upper back to balance the energy along the length of the spine. Remove your hands slowly.

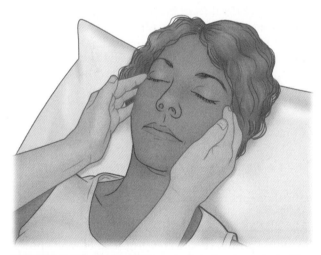

FIGURE 5-27. Head. <u>Light contact circling</u> is applied with the fingertips of both hands over the client's temples.

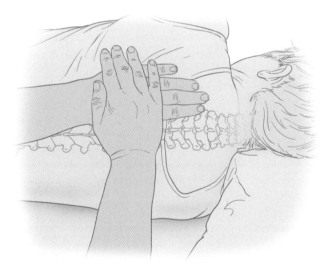

FIGURE 5-28. Back. Apply <u>contact pressure</u> on the erector spinae muscles, lateral to the spine. The left hand is parallel to the spine, and the right hand is used to give added pressure and support. Moving down the back, hold each placement of the hands for approximately 1½ to 2 seconds.

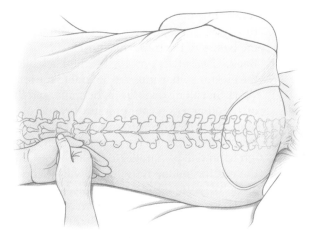

FIGURE 5-29. Low back: Apply <u>broad contact pressure</u> with the back of left hand, using the fist of the right hand to give strength and stability to the press. Let the back of the hand that is in contact be soft, as if gently melting into the client's muscles.

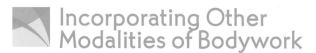

STORY

The Menu

Tim is a massage therapist who participated in the massage program I supervise for hospice. After the initial training he was eager to work with Dennis, a 45-year-old man who had amyotrophic lateral sclerosis (ALS). Dennis was confined to a wheelchair, and while the progression of the disease limited his mobility and his ability to speak, he was mentally alert and receptive to the weekly touch sessions. Tim reported to me that he used the basic techniques of Comfort Touch—encompassing, broad contact pressure, specific contact pressure, and contact circling—for Dennis, while he was seated in his wheelchair. He worked on his head, neck, shoulders, arms, and hands. Dennis was appreciative of this work, indicating, even with his limited ability to speak, his enjoyment of the sessions.

Tim shared with me that he felt it was a privilege to work with Dennis, as he admired the patient's tenacity in spite of living with a debilitating illness. "I have the satisfaction of knowing that I can contribute to the quality of his life."

After several weeks Tim wondered aloud in his conversation with me if there weren't some other techniques he could be using with Dennis. After all, his training in massage school had given him many therapeutic skills from which to choose. He was concerned that he was doing the same thing all the time, saying, "I'm wanting to change or vary the menu for him." I told him that it was okay to continue with the same techniques, if that was what was enjoyable for Dennis. "Some people go

to a restaurant and order something different every week. Others go and find comfort in the familiarity of ordering their favorite meal each time they visit the restaurant. But it is okay to simply ask the client what he wants, letting him know you can adapt to his needs and preferences."

A couple of weeks later, I talked to Tim, who had followed through on my suggestion, telling Dennis that he had some other techniques he could use, if he was interested in trying something different. So Tim had asked him, "What would you like for me to do today?"

Dennis answered, "The usual."

Incorporating Other Modalities of Bodywork

By adhering to the principles of Comfort Touch and using the techniques demonstrated herein, the practitioner can ensure a safe, effective, and satisfying treatment for a very broad range of people. The techniques of Comfort Touch draw from the influences of a number of healing traditions, and the study and practice of these modalities can broaden the range of skills available for the practice of massage with the elderly and the medically frail population. Remember that the primary intention to offer nurturing comfort, rather than to fix or change the individual, remains a hallmark in the practice of Comfort Touch.

Asian Bodywork

Acupressure and Shiatsu are styles of bodywork originating in China and Japan. They are based on an awareness of the flow of life force or **chi** through pathways of energy called **meridians.** Pressure applied to points along these meridians forms the basis for many forms of Asian bodywork. The ancient practice of acupuncture uses fine needles inserted at specific points on the meridians.

The flow of the meridians has some correspondence to the anatomical features recognized in western traditions of medicine, such as the long bones, myofascial networks, and nerve pathways. See Figure 5-30. The 14 major meridians are generally named after an organ with which they have a functional relationship in the theory of traditional Chinese medicine. In addition, some of the major acupressure points that fall along these meridians can be seen to correspond with the **motor points** of muscles. These are areas known to have greater electrical activity. Often found in the belly of a muscle, they correspond to the point where the motor nerve enters the muscle.

meridian (see Figures 5-4, 5-5, and 5-6). The *broad contact pressure* down the legs encompasses the Gallbladder, Stomach, Spleen, and Liver meridians (see Figure 5-18).

Tonic Points

Tonic points are specific acupressure points in the body, known to relieve muscular tension and pain, contribute to relaxation, and promote a sense of well-being. Many of them correspond with the motor points of the muscles. The following are a few of the points that can be incorporated into a Comfort Touch session, enhancing the effectiveness of the work. (Note that all of these points can be used to treat oneself, as well.) Use *specific contact pressure* on the point, holding for a few seconds (or through one respiratory cycle—inhalation and exhalation) before release.

- **Gallbladder-21:** Traditionally referred to as "shoulder well," this point is located in the belly of the trapezius muscle at the top of the shoulder, straight down from the ear (see Figure 5-12). Pressure on this point brings welcome relief for people of all ages and levels of physical condition. Always begin with *broad contact pressure* to warm the area, followed by *specific contact pressure* and *specific contact circling* (see Figure 5-11). Attention to this most significant point has tonifying effects for the entire upper body, as it is a crossover point for the energy meridians and the myofascial network of the head, neck, and shoulders. Pressure exerted here, along with pressure on the acupressure points along the occipital ridge, is very effective in relieving neck pain. It is usually *not necessary or safe* to apply specific pressure into the neck itself.
- **Large Intestine-4:** Located in the web between the thumb and index finger of the hand (see Figure 5-22), this point, along with Large Intestine-10, is used to relieve tension in the hand and lower arm. It is also known to relieve headaches, constipation, and menstrual cramps.
- **Large Intestine-10:** Located in the belly of the brachioradialis muscle (see Figure 5-23), this point, along with Large Intestine-4, is used to relieve tension in the arm and lower arm. It is also known to relieve headaches, constipation, and menstrual cramps.
- **Stomach-36:** Located in the belly of the tibialis anterior muscle of the lower leg, this point is tonifying for the digestive system (see Figure 5-31). *Contact pressure* and *contact circling* on and around this point helps relieve tension and/or fatigue in the legs.
- **Bladder-10 and Gallbladder-20:** These points are located along the occipital ridge at the base

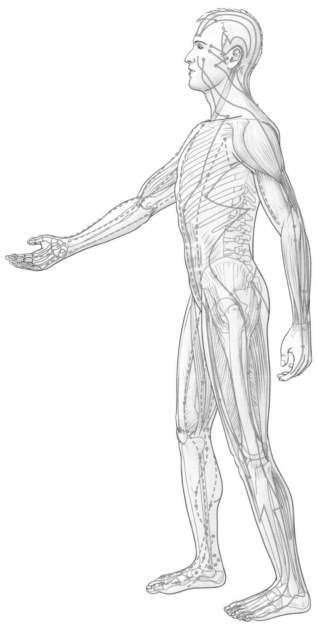

FIGURE 5-30. The meridians of acupressure. The meridians represent complex pathways of <u>chi</u> (energy) in the human body. The meridians shown as solid lines (<u>yang</u>) tend to be on the outer surfaces of the body. These are areas of greater tissue density; whereas, the meridians shown as dotted lines (<u>yin</u>) tend to be on inner, less exposed, and more tender areas of the body. In Comfort Touch the major tonic points are generally located on the <u>yang</u> meridians.

Awareness of Meridians

The individual with training in Asian bodywork will recognize that the sequences of Comfort Touch often follow major meridians. For example, the sequence utilizing *contact pressure* into the erector spinae muscles along the spine, corresponds to the flow of the Bladder

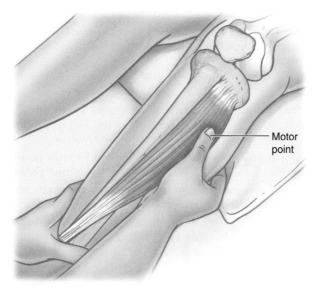

FIGURE 5-31. Tonic point in lower leg—Stomach-36:
Apply specific contact pressure and specific contact circling to the belly (motor point) of the tibialis anterior muscle of the lower leg.

of the skull (see Figure 5-32). The Bladder-10 points are lateral to the midline of the skull approximately 1½ inches apart. These points help relieve eyestrain, tension headaches and neck pain. The Gallbladder-20 points are also located along the occipital ridge, approximately

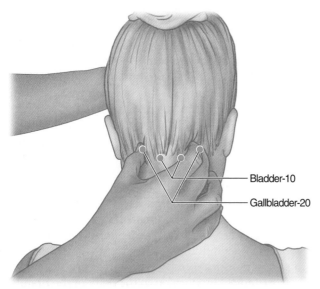

FIGURE 5-32. Tonic points on the occipital ridge—Bladder-10 and Gallbladder-20: Located on the occipital ridge of the skull, the Bladder-10 points are lateral to the mid-line and approximately 1½ inches apart. The Gallbladder-20 points are also located along the occipital ridge, approximately 3 inches apart. Apply specific contact pressure and specific contact circling to these points, using your thumbs and/or the pads of your fingertips.

3 inches apart. They are useful in relieving head, neck, and shoulder pain, and general myofascial tension in the body.

- **Conception Vessel 6:** Located approximately 2 inches below the navel, in the center of the abdomen, this point is also called the "sea of chi" or "sea of energy" (see Figure 5-25). Anatomically, it relates to the organs of the lower digestive tract, and its rich network of nerve plexuses. It is the gravitational center of the body. *Broad contact pressure* over this point is very comforting to the individual, allowing release of deeply held physical and emotional tension. Attention to this point helps facilitate deep, easy, and full breathing. Metaphorically, it corresponds to nurturance and assimilation of experience in the body. It can be thought of as the reservoir of creative energy in the body.
- **Governing Vessel 20:** This point is located at the top of the head, in the soft spot (anterior fontanel) along the midline of the skull. Traditionally called the point of "one hundred meetings," it is thought to be the point of connection to the outer world of the individual, or to the world of spirit. Also called the "all forgiving point," attention to this point helps to balance the right and left sides of the body. Light holding of this point is often used to close a session (see Figure 5-16).

Integrative Massage

Integrative massage is a style of bodywork that acknowledges the relationship of emotional experience and expression to the patterns of myofascial holding (armoring) in the body. Massage is seen as a vehicle to assist the individual in releasing tension in the body resulting from stress and/or trauma. Techniques of this modality are designed to integrate the parts of the body, harmonizing the physical, emotional, mental, and spiritual aspects of the self.

Nurturing in intention, integrative massage uses full hand contact to perform long, slow, gliding strokes that move from the core of the body to the periphery, while overlapping joints to connect body parts. As the practitioner works with an awareness of her or his own fluid body patterning, she or he imparts a quality of ease and flowing energy to the client. The breath is used as a means to foster self-awareness in the client, facilitating release of holding patterns in the body, and engendering openness and expansiveness. By creating a safe and nonjudgmental atmosphere, the integrative massage therapist helps to restore a sense of wholeness and well-being for the client.

Comfort Touch shares a common purpose with Integrative Massage in its intention of offering nurturing relaxation to the individual. Both share an attitude of respect for the integrity of the client as a whole human being. While Comfort Touch is safe for a very broad range of clientele, the specific techniques of Integrative Massage (variations of gliding and kneading) are generally more suitable for a younger and physically healthier population.

Body Energy Therapies

Also called *energy medicine* or *vibrational healing*, **body energy therapies** are modalities that are based on an understanding and/or awareness of subtle energy which surrounds and permeates the human body. This energy is referred to by various names, including biomagnetism, chi, ki, prana, etheric energy, aura field, chakras, and orgone. Body energy therapies derive from many cultural and spiritual healing traditions, including but not limited to Chi Kung, Johrei, Reiki, Therapeutic Touch, Polarity Therapy, Healing Touch, Attunement, and prayer. Techniques involve light touch or hands held a few inches from the body of the client, to influence and balance the energy field. Some modalities focus on areas of the body relating to endocrine glands and/or major organs and nerve plexuses.

Various explanations have been used to describe the mode of action or therapeutic effects of body energy therapies. Scientific study has been done regarding effects to the electromagnetic field of the body.[5] The radiant heat emanating from the hands of the healer may be a direct cause of comfort in the client, as it conducts heat into the body tissues, leading to relaxation. Further study is needed to assess the issues of air flow, and the effects of pressure, movement, and stillness on the nervous system. Other explanations for the healing effects of energy healing rely on traditions based in spiritual beliefs and experiences.

In all of these practices there is an emphasis on the quality of presence and the focused state of mind held by the practitioner. Some practitioners emphasize specific treatment outcomes, while others rely on the intention to assist clients in their own healing process, without specific concern for results.

Most styles of energy work use techniques that involve only light touch or complete non-contact of the client's body. While energy healing modalities have benefit for many, experience in the practice of Comfort Touch, relative to non-contact energy work, demonstrates the preferences of the elderly and the ill to actually be physically touched. Those who are elderly, ill, or disabled may wonder why someone would be hesitant to actually touch them. The sense of isolation among so many people, is most readily ameliorated by the direct physical contact offered through Comfort Touch.

Summary

- The techniques of Comfort Touch are based on the six guiding principles denoted by the word SCRIBE: *slow, comforting, respectful, into center, broad,* and *encompassing.*
- The techniques are often practiced on clients who are fully clothed and may be performed in the seated, supine, or side-lying position.
- The basic techniques of Comfort Touch rely on varying degrees and applications of pressure applied to the body. These include: *encompassing, broad contact pressure, specific contact pressure, broad contact circling,* and *specific contact circling.*
- A variety of other techniques are used to meet the particular needs of the client. These include: *encompassing lift and squeeze, encompassing joint or limb movement, broad contact brushing, holding, water stroke,* and *moisturizing the skin.*
- Comfort Touch is performed on clients in the position that is most comfortable, safe, and appropriate for them. Sequences of touch are presented for the seated position, the supine position, and the side-lying position.
- Comfort Touch is influenced by other traditions of bodywork. Understanding of these modalities can enhance the range of skills available to the practitioner of Comfort Touch. These modalities include Asian bodywork, Integrative massage, and Body Energy Therapies.

Review Questions

1. How does the knowledge of anatomy contribute to the effectiveness of a Comfort Touch session?
2. Why are awareness of the breath and the concept of grounding important for the practitioner of Comfort Touch?
3. How is the principle "into center" applied in the basic techniques of Comfort Touch?
4. How is the principle "broad" applied in the basic techniques of Comfort Touch?
5. How is the principle "encompassing" applied in the basic techniques of Comfort Touch?
6. Give an example where you would use the technique of *encompassing.*

7. Give examples where you would use the techniques of *broad contact pressure* and *specific contact pressure*.

8. Describe the purpose of *specific contact circling*.

9. Give an example where it would be appropriate to use technique of *encompassing lift and squeeze*.

10. Describe how you could incorporate movement into a Comfort Touch session?

11. Which additional technique of Comfort Touch would you use to help relieve edema?

12. Which additional technique of Comfort Touch would you use to apply lotion to dry skin?

13. Which technique may be used as a finishing stroke when completing work on a limb?

14. Which technique is especially appropriate for closing a session?

References

1. Bowden B, Bowden J. *An Illustrated Atlas of the Skeletal Muscles.* 2nd ed. Englewood, CO: Morton Publishing Company; 2005.

2. Netter FN. *Atlas of Human Anatomy.* 4th ed. Philadelphia, PA: Elsevier Health Sciences; 2007.

3. Warfel JH. *The Extremities: Muscles and Motor Points.* Baltimore: Lippincott Williams & Wilkins; 1993.

4. Warfel JH. *The Head, Neck, and Trunk.* Baltimore: Lippincott Williams & Wilkins; 1993.

5. Becker RO, Selden G. *The Body Electric: Electromagnetism and the Foundation of Life.* New York: Harper; 1998.

Suggested Reading

Acland's DVD Atlas of Human Anatomy: The Upper Extremity, The Lower Extremity, The Trunk, The Head and Neck, Part 1, The Head and Neck, Part 2, and The Internal Organs [DVD]. Baltimore: Lippincott Williams & Wilkins; 2003.

Anatomy and Physiology Made Incredibly Easy. 2nd ed. Baltimore: Lippincott Williams & Wilkins; 2005.

Andrade C-K, Clifford P. *Outcome-Based Massage: From Evidence to Practice.* 2nd ed. Baltimore: Lippincott Williams & Wilkins; 2008.

Gach ME. *Acupressure's Potent Points: A Guide to Self-Care for Common Ailments.* New York: Bantam Books; 1990.

Hedley G. *The Integral Anatomy Series, vol. 1: Skin and Superficial Fascia* [DVD]. New Paltz, NY: Integral Anatomy Productions; 2005.

Hedley G. *The Integral Anatomy Series, vol. 2: Deep Fascia and Muscle* [DVD]. New Paltz, NY: Integral Anatomy Productions; 2005.

Lundberg P. *The Book of Shiatsu: A Complete Guide to Using Hand Pressure and Gentle Manipulation to Improve Your Health, Vitality and Stamina.* New York: Simon and Schuster; 2003.

Marieb EN. *Human Anatomy and Physiology.* 7th ed. San Francisco, CA: Benjamin Cummings; 2006.

Rose MK. *Comfort Touch: Massage for the Elderly and the Ill* [Video DVD]. Boulder, CO: Wild Rose; 2004.

Serizawa K. *Effective Tsubo Therapy: Simple and Natural Relief without Drugs.* Tokyo, Japan: Japan Publications; 1984.

Thompson G. *Shiatsu: A Complete Step-by-Step Guide.* New York: Sterling Publishing Company; 1994.

Tortora GJ, Derrickson B. *Principles of Anatomy and Physiology,* 11th ed. Hoboken, NJ: John Wiley and Sons; 2007.

Yamamoto S, McCarty P. *Barefoot Shiatsu.* New York: Avery; 2002.

6

Special Considerations in the Use of Comfort Touch

> **Touch is incredible. You look in the eyes of the patient, knowing you made a difference.**
> **—Kathleen Pressley, PTA**

*W*ith a clear understanding of the principles of Comfort Touch and a foundation in the hands-on skills of this modality, the benefits of touch can be extended to a broad range of people in a variety of settings. This chapter will provide additional information to help the practitioner of Comfort Touch to better serve individuals with special needs.

Comfort Touch is designed to be safe and appropriate for many people, including the elderly and those affected by illness or disability. While it is helpful to study the conditions and pathologies affecting clients in order to adapt to their needs, it is most important to focus on their wholeness as persons. With the respectful attitude and nurturing intention inherent in the practice

of Comfort Touch, the specific needs of the client can easily be accommodated.

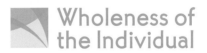

Wholeness of the Individual

Often it is a specific condition, illness or complaint that brings the client—or the client's caregivers—to request massage. In much of health care, it is the complaint or "what is wrong with the person" that is the focus of treatment. In the practice of Comfort Touch, the ailments or limitations of the client are useful to recognize, but it is also wise to acknowledge "what is right with the person." No matter the severity of the patient's condition, it is helpful to emphasize the wholeness of the individual, even in small ways. For example, a patient may be bedridden and unable to

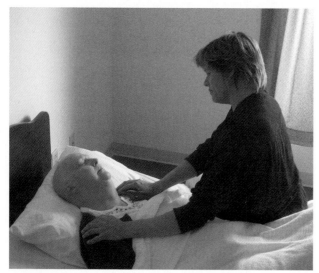

FIGURE 6-1. A woman is comforted by her daughter.
Though living with cancer, this woman is able to enjoy Comfort Touch provided by her daughter.

speak, but she is still able to feel and enjoy touch—to appreciate the warmth of human connection and compassion. (See Figure 6-1.)

Adapting to the Client's Needs

Whenever possible, it is helpful to gather information about a patient's condition before beginning a Comfort Touch session to ensure the safest, most appropriate, and most effective use of techniques. Understanding the pathology of a given disease also allows the practitioner to be more empathetic and understanding of the client's circumstance. But there are times where it is difficult to access information, for example, if the patient is not able to communicate clearly. Even with a detailed medical history of the client, the practitioner of Comfort Touch cannot be expected to be knowledgeable about all the ramifications of many diseases or pathological conditions.

It is important to recognize that there might be a broad variation of symptoms even within a group of people who have the same disease. For example, one person with multiple sclerosis may be very active and mobile, while another with the same disease may have great difficulty in walking. This is true of people with many other diseases and conditions, including diabetes, heart disease, asthma, Parkinson's, etc.

In order to best meet the needs of the client, look at two aspects of the person's condition—*functionality* and levels of *pain* and/or *discomfort*. These two aspects

operate on the physical, mental, and emotional levels of the individual's experience. (See Chapter 2 for more detail on Physical and Psychosocial Issues of the Elderly and the Ill.)

Functionality

Functionality refers to the individual's ability to function in her or his own body, utilizing the physiological capabilities of the body in a normal state or in a healthy adaptation to change. For example, does the person have difficulty breathing? If so, does she or he use supplemental oxygen? The therapist will adapt the body positioning of the client to best accommodate ease of breathing. If a person has limited mobility, the therapist can help her or him or her to get in the most comfortable position for the touch session.

On the *physical* level, functionality can refer to any of a number of factors in the client's experience. Some of these functions include:

- The ability to move and/or the degree of movement in the whole body or any part of the body
- The ability to breathe, with or without supplemental oxygen or the use of a ventilator
- The ability to speak and communicate
- The ability to eat without assistance
- The ability to use the special senses of sight, hearing, taste, and smell
- The control of bowel and bladder functions

If patients are able to communicate, you can assess their level of functionality by asking questions such as, "Are you comfortable in this position? Would you like to move? Is it okay when I move your shoulder?" You can observe their ease of breathing. Notice if they can hear your questions adequately.

On the *mental* level, functionality refers to the cognitive function of the individual. In other words, does the individual understand and process information accurately and appropriately? What is the quality of her or his memory—both long-term and short-term? How does the mental state of the client affect her or his ability to communicate with others and manage everyday living? If there are limitations in mental functioning, the Comfort Touch practitioner will need to be mindful to communicate in a clear and simple manner that is respectful of the client's needs.

On the *emotional* level, functionality refers to the psychological state of the individual. The client may exhibit a full range of emotional expression, from happiness to sadness, from anger to anxiousness. It is *not* the role of the Comfort Touch practitioner to diagnose mental or psychological conditions, but again, she or he may be mindful of this range of expression, and gently accommodate to the client's needs.

Pain and Discomfort

While the various levels of functionality can be observed, pain, as well as its assessment, is a subjective experience. The range of responses to painful stimuli varies greatly from one person to another. Acute pain is the body's voice of warning, alerting the individual to injury in the body. Chronic pain can be the result of one or more factors, including damage to body tissues or organs, inflammation, chronic tension in muscles, or nerve impingement.

The sensation of pain can be modified by many factors, including memory, association, and the anticipation of pain. Some people are tolerant of pain, or have an attitude of "grin and bear it." Others are incapacitated by it. Pain can contribute to an array of emotional responses, including frustration, anger, sadness, depression, and hopelessness.

Surgery may be used to repair tissue injury, thereby treating the underlying causes of some pain. Pharmaceutical drugs are also used to help alleviate pain. However, for many people, the experience of pain persists, and accompanies or contributes to the loss of function. The fear of creating more pain can increase muscular tension, leading to more pain. The anticipation of pain also can inhibit people from physical activity or from moving an affected part of the body, leading to loss of muscle tone and consequent loss of function.

When offering Comfort Touch to people in pain, keep a respectful attitude, trusting your clients' assessments of their own pain. Do not judge them for their response to it. The health care worker who makes a comment like "She couldn't be in that much pain," conveys a disrespectful attitude toward the patient, which can actually interfere with the healing process. Remember that by acknowledging the person's experience, you show your care and concern. The intention inherent in the practice of Comfort Touch allows the patient to relax, sometimes even in spite of the pain. Having something to feel good about *is* an antidote to pain. Caring touch helps to alleviate the fear, anxiety, and depression that often accompany pain. It can break the cycle of pain, offering a change of perspective, a healing distraction from discomfort and suffering.

When beginning a session, ask the client if she or he has any areas of pain or discomfort needing attention. Ask if there are areas you should avoid. Some kinds of pain, such as muscle pain, can be alleviated by the direct pressure of Comfort Touch. With other kinds of pain, such as inflammatory pain due to arthritis, direct pressure would cause more discomfort. (See Precautions in the Use of Touch in Chapter 3.)

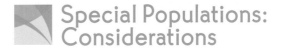

Special Populations: Considerations

There is an apparent simplicity to this modality of touch—an immediacy in the sense of compassion and connection. As the practitioner becomes confident in the application of the specific techniques, deeper layers of intricacy become apparent. Each client brings new information, awareness, challenges, and/or rewards to the practice of Comfort Touch.

Psychological Issues and Trauma

The emotional and physical experiences of each one of us are intertwined and ultimately inseparable. This is the dominant view of holistic medicine, in which the individual is recognized as a whole and multifaceted human being. Touch affects the mental and emotional health of the individual as well as her or his physical body. Modern medicine recognizes the need to address psychological issues, even as it uses an array of substances and methods to address physical ailments and concerns. The practitioner of Comfort Touch needs to be comfortable with the reality of the client's emotional expression, and learn to react in an appropriate and helpful manner.

Remember that it is *not* the job of the Comfort Touch practitioner to diagnose anyone's psychological condition, just as it not within our scope of practice to diagnose physical disease. That is the role of other medical specialists, trained and experienced in diagnostic techniques. However, we may be in a position to provide touch as a complementary therapy to a patient receiving other aspects of medical treatment. People may be referred for massage or Comfort Touch by other health care professionals, who recognize its potential benefit for the patient.

Sometimes, individuals come to us seeking the benefits of touch, and we recognize the need to refer them for additional help from other professionals, whether for treatment by a physician, psychologist, or other appropriate health care provider. If you are working in a medical setting, there will be other people who can help sort out the patient's needs. In a private practice of massage, you can make suggestions, based on your connections with other health care professionals, including psychotherapists and social workers. You can suggest that the client ask for referrals from her or his own family physician.

Adhering to the principles of Comfort Touch, you can provide support to the person suffering from emotional distress, pain, or discomfort associated with acute trauma or traumatic memories.

Hints for Practice

Intuition

Intuition is the process of arriving at a conclusion without having gone through a conscious decision making process. It is the sense of knowing what to do without necessarily knowing why. You might be in a situation and say, "I just knew what to do." Or "I just had a feeling that I should simply hold her hand." Intuition is a very useful ability to develop in the practice of Comfort Touch, as you will frequently encounter situations that require you to be versatile and flexible in your approach with the patient.

Here are three ways to develop your intuition:

1. Experience. Practice your hands-on skills in situations that are relatively predictable and in which you can develop your confidence. For example, practice the techniques of Comfort Touch with a friend or family member, where you can elicit open and honest feedback.

2. Knowledge. Continue your study of anatomy and pathology by reviewing or researching the diseases and conditions that are being experienced by the patients in your care. This increases your knowledge base, and gives a foundation for the insights that arise as you work.

3. Sensation. Most often, intuition is based on the full use of your senses, also called **full sensory perception.** For example, you may intuit that you should place your hands on the client's shoulder, exerting a broad, encompassing pressure. The client's comment, "Oh, how did you know that's just what I needed?" confirms your intuition about placing your hands there as you begin the session. But you actually may have noticed, albeit unconsciously, that the client was holding that shoulder in a rigid, contracted posture. Or you may feel a twinge of discomfort in your own body which corresponds to something that is felt by the client.

Pay attention to all your senses as you work. Notice what you see, for example, in the subtle movements created by the breath as the client is touched. Notice if she or he leans into your touch, or away from it. Feel the texture and temperature of the client's body. Listen to the tone and quality of the individual's voice. Even the sense of smell has information to inform our intuition. And, of course, don't hesitate to ask the client for feedback about what you notice, always respecting the verbal information the individual may share with you.

Emotional Distress

Those who are in physical pain or who have suffered from the loss of function, often struggle with uncomfortable and sometimes conflicting emotions. For example, the patient with a life-threatening illness may be angry about having the disease, or fearful of its progression. She or he can appreciate the care and concern offered by others, while at the same time feeling anxious, frustrated, or despairing. Other feelings may include sadness, guilt, or depression. (See Bereavement—Dealing with Grief and Loss in Chapter 2.)

As practitioners of Comfort Touch, we touch the client's physical body, but we also touch and influence the emotional being. By holding the intention to comfort and the attitude of respect, we allow the individual to be accepting of her or his own feelings. There is no need to judge the emotions as good or bad, positive, or negative. There is no need to try to sort out the feelings or to fix or change them. The input given to the body through nurturing touch does provide opportunity for the client to experience a change of perspective, which in turn allows a change in the experience of otherwise stressful or uncomfortable emotions.

Listening to clients is important, letting them know that you hear what they are saying. For example, you can validate their experience by reflecting back what is said, "Yes, it must be frustrating," or "Yes, it is hard to understand all these changes." Keep your words simple, and avoid projecting your own thoughts or fears onto the situation.

Remember to stay present and grounded in your own body, so that you don't sink into a pit of sympathy with your clients, where you feel as bad as they do. You are most helpful if you stay in a neutral place of compassion, offering your care and concern. In so doing, you offer people a helping hand to assist them out of the depths of their pain and discomfort.

Acute Trauma

Acute trauma is the experience of physical, emotional, or psychic injury in the moment. It could be a momentary crisis resulting from the experience of a painful or uncomfortable medical procedure. It could be an accidental wound, or an emotional shock. Acute trauma can be primarily physical with attendant emotional trauma. Or it may be primarily emotional in nature, such as the shock one experiences at hearing a difficult medical diagnosis for oneself or a loved one.

Sometime you might be the first person to arrive at the scene of an accident. Or you might be present with someone experiencing acute trauma in a medical or homecare setting. It can be disconcerting to find yourself with someone who is expressing deep emotional or physical pain. If you are not comfortable with the expression of feeling yourself, this may add to the challenge. However, with training and experience you can learn to be effective in helping individuals survive and thrive in these situations.

To ensure your effectiveness in supporting the person experiencing acute trauma, pay attention to the following:

- **Physical safety:** If you are the only person available, you need to quickly assess the situation for safety. It is advisable to have training in a Red Cross First Responder course. Keep your own physical safety in mind, then pay attention to the physical safety of others. If necessary, call local emergency services or 911.
- **Stay grounded:** The quality of your presence conveys a sense of safety to the client. Focus on your own sense of connection to the earth beneath you, and you will create an atmosphere that is calming for the client, regardless of the circumstance or emotions being felt and expressed.
- **Stay present:** Focus on what is happening in the present moment, rather than attempting to ignore it or shift attention to the past or present. For example, avoid saying, "Why did this happen?" or "You will feel better tomorrow."
- **Listen and validate:** Listen to what the person is saying and reflect that back. For example, you might say, "Yes, I hear you," or "Tell me exactly how you feel." Avoid saying, "Don't worry. It won't hurt." or "It's not that bad." In other words, do not minimize or invalidate the person's experience, but let her or him know it is okay to talk about it and/or to express feelings.
- **Accept crying as healthy:** The client may express feelings through tears, sometimes subtle, sometimes in a torrent of weeping. It might be appropriate to offer reassurance by saying, "It is okay to cry." Know that the physical act of crying can have a profound healing effect on the body, as it allows pent up energy to be released, much like the release of rain in a thunderstorm. Another lighthearted way to validate the experience of the person who is crying, is to say, "Crying is the body's way of taking a shower from the inside out."
- **Touch simply and directly:** Following the principles of Comfort Touch, take advantage of the power of touch to convey nonverbally a sense of calmness and reassurance. Often it is this touch—slow, broad, encompassing contact—that helps break the cycle of fear that characterizes a traumatic experience. The touch can be as simple as placing a hand on the person's shoulder. Maintain steady contact, avoiding any sudden movements. Consistency of presence and contact convey safety to the person. Respect the person's cues about whether she or he prefers to be touched or not.
- **Allow the client to move into a comfortable position:** Sometimes a person experiencing acute traumatic stress will want to move, trying to find a comfortable position. For example, one may contract one's body, as if moving into a fetal position, or draw the arms together over the chest. Allow the client to move in this manner. You can easily accommodate your touch to the client's movements or positioning, rather than expecting the client to adapt to you, or stay in a position that augments the feeling of vulnerability.
- **Ask appropriate questions:** It may be appropriate to ask, "How can I help?" or "What do you need?" The person might need something as simple as a glass of water, or a tissue to dry teary eyes. Avoid asking, "What's wrong?" as this assumes that one's expression of deep feeling is undesirable.

Traumatic Memories

Sometimes in the practice of bodywork, clients get in touch with deep feelings, evoked by the physical contact to their bodies. As one's body relaxes, memories held locked in the body's nervous system may rise to the surface of consciousness, stirring an emotional response as if the experience was occurring in the present. Touch can act as a catalyst to trigger the release of a range of physical and emotional responses. Your appropriate response can serve as an avenue for healing old wounds. The person may re-experience the past within the context of the safety you provide.

Emotional release does not rid the body of trauma. You cannot extract or delete a memory from the nervous system. But the input of caring touch and compassionate attention gives new information to the nervous system, allowing a change of perspective, a reorganization of information that can empower the individual to live more freely in the present, in spite of events that occurred in the past.

Comfort Touch is often a preferred form of massage for people who have experienced physical or sexual abuse. Because the client can be fully clothed, she or he may feel less vulnerable than with conventional massage, and find it easier to relax while being touched.

To be helpful to the client follow all the guidelines mentioned for working with a client experiencing acute trauma: attend to safety issues; stay grounded and present; listen and validate the individual; keep touch simple and direct, encouraging comfortable body positioning; ask for feedback on how you can help. Here are some additional guidelines:

- **Normalize feelings:** Let the clients know by your response that you are not judging them. Sometimes when people experience emotional release they feel not only the emotions associated with the past trauma (ie, shock, anger, fear), but they feel guilty, embarrassed, or apologetic about having an outburst of emotion. Through your attitude you convey a sense of acceptance, validating that it is normal and healthy for the individual to express feelings, thereby releasing their hold on the body.

- **Empower the person, not the trauma:** Focus on the wholeness of the person, validating her or his expression. You comfort the person by focusing on her or his inner strength and resources. Focus on the ability to survive the trauma, rather than on the trauma itself.

- **Speak the person's name and reference the body's experience:** When addressing the person in great emotional distress, it can be helpful to use her or his name. For example, say, "Helen, tell me what you are feeling now in your body." Acknowledging the person by name can help to keep her or him in the present. Asking about sensations in the body can help to keep her or him connected to the body, rather than disconnecting from it or withdrawing into the past. Memories relate to experiences of the past, but healing and integration occur in the present moment, by accepting the body and reality as it is now.

- **Remember to breathe and stay grounded:** Maintain your own sense of grounding. Breathe deeply and fully. If you do this as you touch the person, it will remind him or her to breathe also, allowing integration of emotions and physical sensations in the body.

- **Know when to refer:** Remember that it is your role to comfort, not to psychoanalyze the client. You may need to refer the individual for professional mental health counseling or services.

Infants and Children

Infants and children are a very special population who can benefit from Comfort Touch. Practitioners can help them through the direct application of specific techniques of touch. They can also assist the parents to feel more confident and effective in the use of touch with their own children.

Supporting Parent/Child Relationships With Touch

Massage with infants and children is primarily the role of the parents. From the first encompassing hugs of a mother for her newborn baby, to the reassuring contact offered to a child in need, touch is a means of nurturing a developing human being. (See Figure 1-1.) The conscious use of touch can be used in everyday tasks, such as dressing or bathing the young child. For example, the basic techniques of broad, encompassing contact pressure can be used when applying lotion or oil after the baby's bath, as shown in Figure 6-2.

Parents instinctively use the Comfort Touch principles of *broad* and *encompassing* contact as they hold their children. (See Figure 6-3.) The quality of presence and grounding of the adult, coupled with this instinctive and natural way of holding the child, allows the child in distress to relax. In this relationship the touch is mutually comforting and enjoyable for both parent and child.

Addressing Needs of Infants and Children

The principles of Comfort Touch and the inherent adaptability of this modality make it suitable to meet the needs of infants and children. The child can be

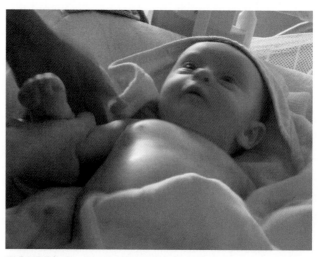

FIGURE 6-2. Comforting infant massage. The parent of this infant uses broad encompassing contact to apply lotion after the baby's bath.

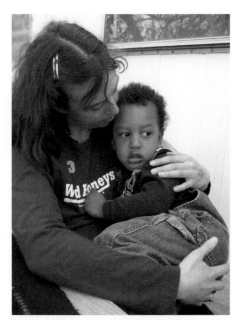

FIGURE 6-3. A mother comforts her child. A parent instinctively follows the principles of Comfort Touch when she holds a child with broad, encompassing contact.

fully clothed and no special equipment or lotion is required. Often only a few minutes of touch are needed to elicit a positive response. An infant or small child can be held in the arms, while sitting in the lap of the Comfort Touch practitioner for a short session, using *specific contact pressure* on tonic acupressure points. (See Chapter 5.)

It is helpful to have a playful attitude when working with infants and children. Maintain eye contact and respond to their moving bodies, rather than try to hold them in a rigid position. Be especially sensitive to their physical responses and feedback, stopping or pausing as they adjust to your touch. If your contact is enjoyable to them, they will allow you to continue, even when they are initially in distress, for example, with respiratory congestion or colic.

The following are considerations in the use of Comfort Touch with infants and children:

- **Newborn infants:** The newborn infant is stimulated and comforted by touch. The Comfort Touch practitioner can help to ease the trauma of birth through the broad encompassing contact of *general contact pressure*. This touch is warming for the newborn, and helps to facilitate the sense of bonding connection. The new parents of the infant can be encouraged to touch and hold the baby. In some instances, where the child has hypertonic (tense) muscles, *broad contact pressure* and *specific contact pressure* can be used to facilitate relaxation of the muscles.

In hypotonic (low tone) muscles, *contact circling* can be used to stimulate circulation and nerve response to increase tone. This may be especially helpful to the newborn who is born with limp muscles, regardless of the cause. In this situation the baby may be in a specially heated bassinet, under warming lights. The massage therapist who is experienced in perinatal massage can use the techniques of Comfort Touch, in this circumstance, working cooperatively under the supervision of the obstetric physician and/or nurses.

- **Babies:** Comfort Touch can be used with babies, not only for general stimulation and relaxation, but to treat specific common ailments. For example, *general* and *specific contact pressure* can be applied to the baby's feet to help alleviate indigestion and/or colic. The baby can be held in the practitioner's arms or she or he may be lying down on a padded surface. (See Figure 6-4.) *Specific contact pressure* on the foot, and especially the toes, can relieve sinus congestion or respiratory distress. Work slowly, watching the baby's reaction. As you encompass the foot, move with the baby's overall movement.

- **Children:** Most children do not have the same degree of tension in the musculature as adults; therefore, they respond to touch much quicker than adults. They also have a much shorter attention span, so keep hands-on sessions relatively short and focused on the area of greatest tension or pain (ie, the shoulders or back). When working with children, it is wise to have the parents observe the session, so the child does not feel uncomfortable with being touched by a

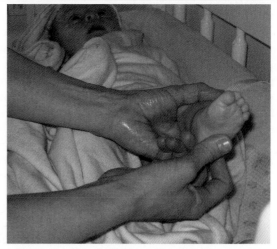

FIGURE 6-4. Contact pressure on a baby's foot. Specific contact pressure is used on the baby's foot to help relieve colic, sinus congestion, or respiratory distress.

non-family member. Doing so also encourages the parents to feel more confident in offering the benefits of touch to their own children.

- **Children and illness:** Illness presents a special opportunity to offer the benefits of Comfort Touch to the child. Often even parents are afraid to touch a child who is not feeling well. Remember that the intention to comfort is reassuring to the child, creating a feeling of safety, which facilitates healing. If a child is in acute distress, *broad contact pressure* and *specific contact circling* along the spine are especially helpful. The child may be in the side-lying position. *Broad contact pressure* on the sacrum is especially calming and grounding for the child.
- **Children with special needs:** The techniques of Comfort Touch are easy to adapt for the child with special needs (eg, a child who is in a wheelchair or has difficulty communicating). Therapists report success with autistic children and children with attention deficit hyperactivity disorder. The slow rhythm and the broad compression of Comfort Touch contribute to its effectiveness for these children.

Perinatal and Postpartum

Comfort Touch is a wonderful complementary therapy providing physical and psychological benefits to support women throughout their pregnancies and birthing experiences. Comfort Touch practitioners who wish to attend births should pursue training (eg, prenatal classes or **doula** birth assistant training), to prepare them to know what to expect as they assist in birth.

Pregnancy

The particular needs of the pregnant woman require that the therapist be versatile in working with her, helping her to find the most comfortable position to receive bodywork. The side-lying position allows easy access to massage the back, and is generally very comfortable for the woman. A pillow is placed under the head, ensuring that the head is in alignment with the back. A pillow is placed between the legs, to ease strain on the low back and hips. The client may hug a pillow for support. A small towel can be placed under the low back if support is needed there. (See Figure 6-5.)

Pregnancy puts added strain on the muscles of the back, especially the low back. Various techniques of Comfort Touch can be used on the back in the side-lying position. See Chapter 5 for the sequence of touch in the side-lying position. Use *broad* and *specific contact pressure* on the erector muscles on either side of the

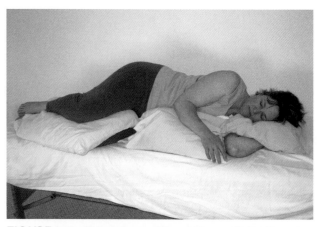

FIGURE 6-5. Side-lying position. Using multiple pillows to support the woman's body, the side-lying position is the preferred position to massage a pregnant woman.

spine. (See Figures 5-28 and 5-29.) Use *specific contact circling* to areas of particular tension. Work closely with the woman's feedback, as she directs you in meeting her needs.

Pressure on the sacrum can help also relieve the low back pain that often accompanies pregnancy. The body can also be gently rocked in this position to alleviate tension along the spine. (See Figure 6-6.) This technique can also be used during labor, helping the woman to relax and rest between contractions.

Labor

During labor the practitioner must be prepared to adapt to the changing needs of the laboring woman. She might want to be touched one moment, and refuse

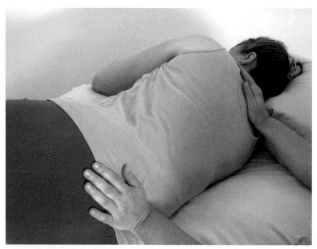

FIGURE 6-6. Side-lying position—sacrum press. Apply firm contact pressure to the sacrum with the woman in the side-lying position.

to be touched the next. Always respect her desires in the moment, letting her know you are available to accommodate her preferences.

In addition to the side-lying position, techniques of Comfort Touch can be applied as the woman is sitting, standing, or squatting. They can be used between contractions to help her to rest. Sometimes firm supporting *contact pressure* is applied to the low back or sacrum during a contraction. During the pushing phase of delivery, touch can be used to give support, helping to keep the woman energized and focused. Massage of the legs and feet is sometimes helpful between pushes, to prevent cramping of the muscles.

During birth, the Comfort Touch practitioner becomes part of a team that is committed to a safe and joyful birth experience. Keep safety uppermost in mind, as you work cooperatively with others, letting your grounded and unobtrusive presence support not only the mother, but her spouse/partner and the medical personnel.

Postpartum

Following the birth, you may have the opportunity to massage the newborn baby. (See the previous section.) Comfort Touch can be used on the mother immediately following the birth, or in the hours and days ahead, depending on her need and your availability. It is a wonderful service to provide the new mother, as she adapts to the changes in her body and the demands of taking care of the new baby.

Medical/Surgical

Comfort Touch has a very broad range of application in the care of medical and surgical patients. Because it is based on the premise that touch is an integral aspect of wellness and the healing process, its benefits can be applied safely, appropriately, and effectively for anyone who is open to being touched. The following are considerations for working with people affected by different illnesses and conditions. This is, by no means, a complete listing. The Comfort Touch practitioner is always reminded to adhere to the principles outline by SCRIBE when encountering new situations. Remember that there might be more variation of symptoms among people who have the same disease as there is among those with different diseases. Also, many people are coping with multiple conditions or diseases.

Acute Illness or Injury

Acute illnesses include anything from the common cold to a sudden heart attack. Common sense will dictate the wisdom of touch in acute medical situations.

Obviously, if the illness or injury is life threatening, you would call your local emergency services (911 phone alert system) to see that the person gets immediate help and transportation to a medical facility, if needed. Short of a life threatening emergency, or if in doubt about the appropriate course of action, call for medical assistance or advice.

In these situations, Comfort Touch has a place. The reassurance of touch to someone in an acute emergency or medical crisis—whether in a medical setting, or outside of it—can keep the person calm until further help arrives. Training in Comfort Touch, with its emphasis on quiet presence and grounding, is a complement to training in first response and emergency care.

All too often in our culture people let their fears of illness keep them from offering a comforting touch to someone who is in pain, or suffering from illness. Friends come to visit someone in the hospital and stand idly by, afraid to touch the one who is sick, for fear of hurting the patient or of catching the illness. Except for rare instances where quarantine is required, a simple touch—just holding a hand or encompassing the feet—can provide the healing balm to help the sick individual feel more confident about recovering from the illness.

Pre- and Postsurgery

Touch can provide comforting reassurance to a patient who is anticipating surgery. A nurturing massage before a scheduled surgery can provide the patient with time to relax and let go of fears about the impending operation. Nurturing contact from a family member, massage therapist, or other health care provider can set an upbeat and positive tone. It is useful to share even a few minutes of Comfort Touch with the patient as she or he is being prepared for admittance to the operating room.

If the surgery is scheduled ahead of time (ie, not an emergency procedure) the patient can discuss this option to have Comfort Touch before the procedure. Consultation with the anesthesiologist can be helpful to ensure that everyone is working to support the best outcome for the patient.

After surgery, the patient is returned to a recovery room. Once approval is given allowing visitors, Comfort Touch is again a helpful option, whether given by family member or another member of the health care team. Extreme caution is observed to touch only the most accessible part of the body. *Stay away from the general area of the surgery.* Avoid motion to the body, and keep touch to simple *broad contact*, using only enough pressure to let the patient know you are there and present to provide support.

Recovery from surgery varies widely depending on the particular surgery and the state of the patient's general health. If the patient is conscious (eg, following outpatient surgery), she or he may only be in recovery for a few hours before returning home. Touch can help to relax muscles that have become tense during the procedure (eg, the shoulder muscles). Keep the touch simple, listening to the patient's feedback. Sometimes, just sitting down and holding the patient's hands or feet is all that is needed.

In more complex surgeries, and/or where general anesthesia is used, it can take several hours for the patient to regain consciousness. Even so, it can be helpful to simply touch the patient. Many who have been in seemingly unresponsive conditions have reported the value of knowing that someone was there present with them. Just because someone cannot speak does not mean she or he cannot hear or feel or appreciate the presence of people who care.

One man who was on a ventilator and sedated for several days after a complex heart surgery later described his experience during the days following his surgery: *"I was on a boat. It was hot and there was no ventilation. The boat was moving. I could hear voices. I wondered why everyone was ignoring me . . . I wondered why no one came to visit me."* Recovery from surgery can be a very isolating, fearful, and disorienting experience. The simplest techniques of Comfort Touch can be used to help in the hours and days following surgery to assist in the healing process.

While blood is pumped via the mechanism of the heart, movement of the lymph is dependent on muscular movement. The broad compression that characterizes Comfort Touch is useful to help encourage the circulation of lymph after someone has been confined to bed for any length of time. (This is why compression hose are used following surgery to assist with circulation in the legs of both blood and lymph.) *Contact pressure* on the feet can help stimulate nerve response, both energizing and relaxing the patient.

The Comfort Touch practitioner working with a postoperative patient will work closely with medical personal to ensure the safety and comfort of the patient. Here are some factors to consider:

- **Cooperate with staff:** Communicate clearly with staff about your intention to comfort the patient. Respect their time and be as unobtrusive as possible. Most hospital staff will welcome family and/or well-meaning visitors (including you as the massage therapist).
- **Practice good hygiene:** Be diligent about handwashing. In some cases you will be required to wear a face mask to limit the spread of airborne pathogens. Check with nursing staff to see if there are any other restrictions.
- **Be careful of medical equipment:** Do not interfere with medical equipment. Take care not to touch any tubing or medical devices attached to the patient.
- **Listen to the patient:** Respond to the patient's needs and feedback regarding the touch you provide.
- **Avoid the site of surgery or pain:** Avoid the site of the surgery itself, and the surrounding tissue. Avoid causing any movement that could contribute to pain. Avoid touching areas of pain, without explicit permission from the patient's doctor.
- **Watch for deep vein thrombosis:** This is a potentially life threatening complication that sometimes follows surgery. It is a blood clot that develops in a deep vein, usually in the leg. This can happen if the vein is damaged or if the flow of blood slows down or stops. It can cause pain in the leg and lead to complications if it breaks off and travels via the bloodstream to the lungs. In some postoperative instances massage will not be allowed below the waist. This is something to be aware of even several weeks post surgery. Avoid deep work on the legs, especially if the patient reports specific pain in the legs. If you suspect this condition, *do not hesitate* to report it to the patient's doctor, so that it can be monitored and proper medical attention directed to the patient's condition.
- **Be respectful and inclusive of others:** Often when providing Comfort Touch in a medical setting you will have other people in the room, either other family members and friends of the patient or medical personnel. Be respectful of their presence, as it need not interfere with the touch you are providing. As you provide the hands-on care to the client, the healing essence of that touch can be seen and felt by others who are present, even if they only visit briefly. The restful atmosphere is tangible to others, and helps them to appreciate the value of the service provided by massage therapists in the medical setting.

Rehabilitation

Rehabilitation is a time of adjusting to changing life circumstances following illness, injury, and/or surgery. It can entail a relatively short amount of time, for example, several days or weeks in a medical setting or outpatient clinic to regain strength and function following surgery. Or it may be a long-term process requiring extensive medical treatment or physical therapy after a life changing event such as a cerebral vascular accident (stroke), spinal cord injury, or traumatic brain injury. Massage can play a significant role in helping the patient cope with the physical and emotional challenges in the process of healing and/or adapting to change. It can bring relief to the patient by addressing specific areas of pain or tension in the body. It also provides the opportunity to encourage the patient in her or his recovery.

In working with the person undergoing rehabilitation keep the following considerations in mind:

- **Collaboration with health care team:** Remember that massage and Comfort Touch provide therapy that is complementary to other treatments including: surgery, pharmaceutical medicine, and physical therapy. The patient might also be receiving occupational therapy, speech therapy, or respiratory therapy. It is your job to work cooperatively with other members of the patient's health care team who are committed to the patient's recovery. Many of these other therapies involve concentration and/or physical focusing of energy, so it is most helpful to let the touch therapy be a time of complete relaxation.

- **Positioning of patient:** As always with Comfort Touch, you can work on the patient in whatever position is most comfortable to him or her, whether in bed, a recliner or a wheelchair. Some wheelchairs can be tilted backward, providing a comfortable position for the patient, without necessitating transfer to a bed. (See Figure 6-7.)

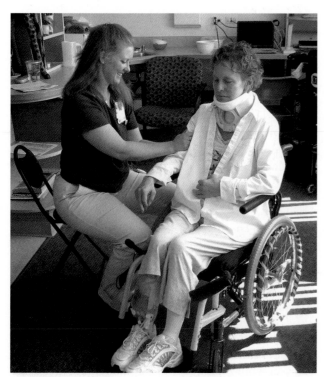

FIGURE 6-7. Comfort Touch in a rehabilitation setting. A nurse helps the patient to relax by using broad encompassing pressure.

- **Patient's tolerance:** Depending on the circumstances for which people are undergoing rehabilitation, their needs for touch will vary. For example, if the patient is very frail, only the gentlest of touch will be needed. If, on the other hand, the patient has a basically strong constitution and is recovering from an injury, she or he may be working very hard (eg, in physical therapy), and will appreciate contact that gives more specific and deeper pressure. Another example is the patient who has suffered a spinal cord injury, paralyzing the lower body. In the process of learning to adapt to navigating via a wheelchair, the muscles of the upper back, shoulders, and arms can become very hypertonic and sore. You can use deeper *general contact pressure* and *specific contact pressure*, and *contact circling*, based on the client's feedback.

- **Sensory perception and motor function:** Paralysis is loss of motor and/or sensory function to any part of the body. It can be caused by a number of factors, including spinal cord injury, stroke, brain tumor, or neuropathy. Assess the patient's level of motor function and sensation before beginning a touch session. She or he will be able to give feedback most easily where sensory function is intact. Generally, touch will be most enjoyable on the parts of the body where the patient has feeling. But it can be useful to parts of the body with loss of motor and sensory function because of the benefits to the circulatory and lymphatic systems.

- **Special needs of patients with traumatic brain injuries:** These injuries are the result of externally applied forces to the brain, caused by motor vehicle accidents, falls, sports injuries, gunshot wounds, or physical violence. They can result in cognitive impairment, changes in motor function, changes in emotional response, and/or behavioral function. In touching these people, keep in mind all the issues of working with patients who have experienced trauma. The person may be very sensitive to touch. She or he may be fearful of touch, especially to the head. Communicate your intentions carefully, work very slowly, and respond to the patient's feedback. Begin with short sessions, for example, by massaging the feet, to see how the person responds. In time, the steady, predictable nature of Comfort Touch can help people with these injuries to relax and enjoy new and healing input to their bodies.

Chronic Illnesses

Comfort Touch can be a valuable part of ongoing complementary care for those living with chronic illnesses.

The benefits of touch can help alleviate the emotional and physical pain and discomfort associated with many diseases.

Cardiac and Pulmonary (Respiratory) Illnesses

Heart disease is the leading cause of death in this country. Cancer, cerebrovascular disease (stroke), and chronic lower respiratory diseases follow in number. As expected, these conditions are prevalent in the elderly population. A combination of genetic predisposition, lifestyle factors, and medical care influence the progression of these illnesses. Diseases affecting the functionality of the heart and lungs include **coronary artery disease**, **congestive heart failure**, **atherosclerosis**, hypertension (high blood pressure), **chronic obstructive pulmonary disease (COPD)**, emphysema, and asthma. Patients range from high functioning and ambulatory to those who are bedridden and require continuous nursing care.

Cardiopulmonary diseases present with a range of symptoms including: fatigue, muscle weakness, shortness of breath, chest pain, coughing, and wheezing. Depression is common in people suffering from heart and lung diseases. Mental functioning may be affected owing to insufficient blood flow to the brain. The causes of heart disease stem from one of the following: inadequate coronary blood supply (eg, due to buildup of fatty deposits in arterial walls); anatomical disorders, such as defective valves; or faulty electrical conduction (arrhythmia) in the heart. The symptoms of lung disease can result from; allergic reaction (bronchial asthma), infection (tuberculosis, pneumonia), cancer, inflammation (bronchitis), or structural changes in the lungs. The term **chronic obstructive pulmonary disease** (COPD) refers to those disorders in which there is some degree of obstruction of the air passages: bronchial asthma, bronchitis, and emphysema.

The function of the heart and lungs are interconnected through their complex and vital functions of blood circulation and respiration. In working with people challenged by heart and lung diseases keep the following in mind:

- **Breathing and oxygen:** Patients with compromised pulmonary function might have external oxygen tanks, with tubing to deliver oxygen via the nose. Be careful not to interfere with the flow of the oxygen. You may need to help reposition the tubing if necessary.
- **Positioning of the client:** Position the client to optimize breathing. Generally it is easier for the client to breathe with the back in a relatively elevated or upright position. The seated position, with the client in a wheelchair or recliner, is comfortable for many. If the patient is in a regular bed, pillows can be used to elevate the back and head. Hospital beds can be adjusted to tilt the patient's back to a more upright posture. Check with patients to get their feedback. (Remember that the prone position is *not* used in the practice of Comfort Touch, in a medical setting. Even for a healthy individual it can be more difficult to breathe while prone.)
- **Edema:** Edema, the accumulation of fluid in the tissues of the extremities, is common. Be careful not to use too much pressure over areas of swelling. In early stages of diseases, use of the *water stroke* (see Figure 5-17) or techniques of manual lymph drainage can be helpful, but in later stages, these techniques will have little effect. Be attentive to the client's feedback, and keep your intention clear to offer comfort, rather than to treat specific symptoms, such as edema or poor circulation.
- **Fragility of blood vessels:** People with cardiopulmonary diseases often have very fragile blood vessels, and therefore are prone to bruising easily. In elderly clients in general, the skin becomes thinner and less elastic, so the fine capillaries beneath the surface have even less protection from pressure. Be especially careful to keep contact pressure broad. Avoid specific pressure applied via the thumb or fingertips.

Cancer

With advances in medical care and treatment, more people are living with and surviving the diagnosis of cancer. Cancer can affect any part of the body, and treatment options include surgery, chemotherapy, and radiation. From the initial stages of diagnosis, through treatment and recovery, touch therapies can provide comforting relief for the individual. For those who do not respond to treatment, Comfort Touch can be part of palliative and hospice care. (See Figure 6-8.)

As you work with people diagnosed with cancer, remember that it is your job to support them in a caring, nonjudgmental manner no matter the course of the disease or their chosen medical treatment options. The person may be overwhelmed by the ramifications of the disease itself, and/or the array of healing modalities presented to them. The massage session is a time to relax and take a break from the fear, uncertainty, and worry that may haunt them everyday. It is a time to feel good in the body, enjoying the pleasures of touch.

When offering Comfort Touch to someone who has undergone surgery, observe the usual precautions that you would with a surgical patient. Avoid the site of the surgery, giving the tissue ample time to heal. Radiation can cause burns to the surface of the skin, so avoid touching it as you would any site of a burn.

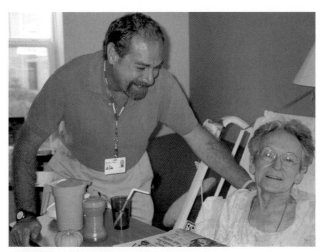

FIGURE 6-8. A woman in a hospice care center. The cheerful attitude and reassuring touch of the health care worker puts this patient at ease in the palliative care setting.

Chemotherapy, which is designed to destroy the growth of cancerous cells, contributes to a range of possible side effects, including: nausea, fatigue, constipation, bruising, skin sensitivity, pain, moodiness, and depression. Other medications to counteract these effects might be given to the patient (eg, anti-nausea drugs), and can help support the patient to a quicker recovery from chemotherapy. Comforting touch helps the patient to relax during the process, which can be prolonged over many weeks, allaying some of the fatigue and psychoemotional aspects of undergoing this kind of medical treatment.

Edema is often present in patients with cancer. Swelling can be found in any part of the body, but it is often most noticeable in the extremities. In the early stages of the disease, techniques of manual lymph drainage or use of the *water stroke* can be helpful to reduce swelling. In later stages of cancer, the functioning of the lymphatic system deteriorates, making it counterproductive to attempt to reduce the swelling through touch. In fact, touch to the edematous part of the body can be very painful. Sometimes gentle massage of the feet can be relaxing, even when touch to swollen ankles would be painful.

Cancer patients vary in the degree of pain they experience, depending on the site of the cancer and the stage of its development. Because pain medicine is an important aspect of medical care, particularly in long-term or terminal cases of cancer, it is important to assess its effects on the patient's ability to give you feedback relative to the amount of pressure you use. Generally you avoid working on the specific site of tumors, areas of swelling, or anywhere that touch could contribute to more pain.

Patients might have specific areas of pain or muscle tension. Listen and respond to their stated needs for bodywork. For general relaxation, the techniques of Comfort Touch can be applied to any and all areas of the body. Many patients respond favorably to work on the hands or the feet, as this helps to calm and relax the whole body.

Diabetes

Since the discovery of insulin in the 1920s and subsequent advances in medical treatment, people with diabetes have been able to live long, healthy, and productive lives. Treatment of the disease requires diligence to avoid the myriad complications that affect the quality of life for diabetics. In the elderly population, diabetes is a disease that is often seen concurrently with other health conditions such as heart disease, stroke, or high blood pressure and kidney disease. Massage and Comfort Touch provide relief from the symptoms and help support diabetics in coping with the everyday challenges that accompany the disease.

Levels of functionality and pain vary widely, ranging from the active, athletic individual, to the one suffering from severe complications of the disease. Consequently, the approach to massage will vary. When functionality is high, clients can receive the bodywork of their choice and benefit from the myofascial and stress reducing effects of massage, which can be part of their regular health care regimens. For frail clients and/or those suffering from complications, Comfort Touch can provide safe and effective relief from pain and discomfort.

Most people affected by diabetes have a genetic disposition to one of the following types:

- **Type 1 diabetes** (insulin dependent diabetes mellitus, or IDDM): Affecting 5 to 10 percent of diabetics, insulin producing cells of the pancreas are damaged or destroyed. Consequently, the individual is dependent on insulin from either regular injections or use of an insulin pump. Though it is a genetic disease, the onset may be triggered by physical or emotional stress. It tends to develop at an earlier age than Type 2 diabetes, but age is not the determining factor for diagnosis.
- **Type 2 diabetes** (non-insulin dependent diabetes mellitus, or NIDDM): Affecting approximately 90 percent of total diabetics, it is more prevalent in people over the age of 40. In these people, the pancreas is producing insulin, but the cells that use insulin are resistant to it. Type 2 diabetics may take oral medications designed to decrease insulin resistance or to enhance the cells' sensitivity to insulin. Some also need to take insulin. Often lifestyle measures, such as

losing weight and/or increasing exercise, improve insulin's efficiency.

In working with people with diabetes, keep the following issues in mind.

- **Myofascial effects:** Physiological changes, including elevated blood sugars, cause a thickening of connective tissue in the diabetic individual, which in turn affects mobility and elasticity of the myofascial system. This can be noted in general levels of stiffness in the muscles, tendons, and ligaments, as well as decreased range of motion in the joints. Stress hormones also contribute to chemical changes in the connective tissue, causing a stickiness between the layers of fascia. Touch therapies can significantly counter this effect. Massage works directly with the muscles and connective tissues in the body, helping to facilitate greater mobility in the body. Work slowly, allowing gentle movement according to the client's preference. The warmth of full hand contact, which emphasizes contact with the palmar surface of the hand, can bring soothing relief to stiff muscles and fascia. Gentle range of motion exercises and stretching can help encourage flexibility and health of the myofascial system.

- **Testing and injection sites:** Specialized meters and test strips are used daily (up to 10 times a day) to monitor blood glucose levels. Adjustments to caloric intake and use of medications are based on these tests. Because most of these tests involve poking the fingertips, they can become very tender or callused. Sensitively applied touch to the fingertips can be beneficial and enjoyable for the client. Generally, it is safe to massage the site of an insulin injection. Occasionally, there might be localized bruising, so respond to the client's feedback to avoid discomfort. Increasingly, more diabetics inject insulin via an insulin pump, a battery-driven device that pumps insulin via a small tube into the abdominal wall. Be careful to avoid pressure on the site itself. Also avoid pulling or pressing on the tubing.

- **Peripheral neuropathy:** Diabetes can lead to damage of the nerves of the hands, arms, feet, and/or legs resulting in numbness, pain, and/or weakness. When touching areas that are affected use caution to prevent pain or discomfort. Avoid touching these areas if they are painful. Use only *broad, encompassing contact pressure,* as it minimizes the danger of causing irritation, and it can bring relief. Many diabetics have extremely ticklish feet. You can also work through socks on the feet to minimize ticklishness.

- **Tissue damage, ulcers:** Because of impaired circulation, diabetics are more prone to tissue damage and slow healing of wounds, particularly to the extremities. Avoid any pressure on sores, open wounds, or areas of bruising. For complications involving ligaments, tendons, or joints, avoid using deep pressure or excessive movement.

- **Hypoglycemia: Hypoglycemia** is the condition in which the individual experiences blood sugar levels below 70 mg/dl. Diabetics vary in their level of awareness and ability to recognize symptoms of hypoglycemia, *which is a very serious and potentially life-threatening condition.* For those using insulin, blood glucose levels should be tested before receiving a massage. Blood glucose levels can change during a session, so it is also important to test after the session. While a moderate drop of 20 to 30 mg/dl can be anticipated, changes in either direction of up to 100 mg/dl have been recorded from one hour to the next.[1,2]

Because of the frequently unpredictable nature of diabetes, it is important to recognize the signs and symptoms of hypoglycemia:

Excessive sweating (skin may feel clammy)
Faintness or headache
Inability to awaken
Spaciness—the person may talk or move slowly, or not be able to speak coherently. (*This may be confused with the more typical relaxed state that one experiences after a massage.*)
Irritability
Change in personality
Rapid heartbeat

If the client shows any of the above signs, ask her or him: "How do you feel?" Note the coherence of the response. Be aware that blood-sugar level can drop quickly, so that treatment must be given *immediately.* If sugars are low, the diabetic needs sugar fast! This may be in the form of fruit juice, honey, a sugary drink, or glucose tablets. (Many diabetics carry their own glucose tablets, or another source of quick-acting carbohydrates, such as juice or candy.) A cup of juice, or the equivalent of 15 to 20 grams of carbohydrates, will usually be sufficient to raise the blood glucose to a safe level. Changes will be noted in the person within minutes, who should be allowed to rest for 10–20 minutes, then encouraged to test her or his blood-glucose level again to see if more carbohydrate calories are needed.

Infectious Diseases

Infectious diseases present special concerns to ensure the safety of both the touch therapist and the patient. Infectious diseases include a broad spectrum of illnesses, from generally short-term conditions such as the common cold, to acute influenza, to long-term chronic diseases such as Hepatitis C or HIV/AIDS. **Septicemia** is a dangerous systemic disease caused by the spread of microorganisms and their toxins via the circulating blood.

People who are elderly and/or suffering from chronic illness (eg, cardiopulmonary diseases) may be especially vulnerable to infection (eg, respiratory infections or staph infections) owing to weakening of the immune system. In the medical setting, there is greater potential for the spread of infection, so care must be maintained when touching patients to observe the good rules of hygiene. (See Chapter 3.)

Patients with infectious diseases are often physically and emotionally isolated from others. The physical isolation may be necessary, especially in acute situations where medical needs must be assessed and treated. The social and emotional isolation can be a very difficult aspect of the illness. But with medical supervision and permission, and observing necessary rules of hygiene and universal precautions, these patients can enjoy the benefits of touch. Always consult with the patient's health care providers before working with this population.

In working with people with known or potentially contagious diseases, consider the following:

- **Hygiene.** Observe all rules of hygiene, including standard and universal precautions. Wash hands carefully before and after touching the patient.
- **Masks.** If patients have respiratory infections, or if there is danger of you infecting them, you may be advised or required to wear a mask. This is often the case in working with post surgical patients, as well. Make sure you are using the mask correctly.
- **Gloves.** In some instances you may be required to wear gloves. For example, you can wear gloves if the patient has a contagious rash, or rash of unknown origin. Generally, you would avoid touching these areas, but if touch would be beneficial, e.g., massage of the feet, you can use broad encompassing pressure, even while wearing gloves for the patient's benefit.

Acquired Immune Deficiency Syndrome (AIDS) is a disease caused by the **human immunodeficiency virus (HIV)** which attacks the immune system, leaving the person vulnerable to a host of opportunistic infections and cancers. It is transmitted from person to person via bodily fluids (blood, semen, vaginal fluid, breast milk). It is not spread via sweat, tears or saliva. Symptoms can be mild to severe, and affect all systems of the body. They include: fatigue, weight loss, fevers, persistent infections, skin rashes, memory loss, respi-

ratory distress, lack of coordination, gastrointestinal distress, headaches, hypertension, muscular tension, and neuropathy. Because of advances in medical treatment, many people living with this once fatal infection can now live relatively healthy and productive lives for many years after diagnosis.

Massage can provide the physical benefits of general neuromuscular relaxation, along with the psychoemotional benefits of safe and comforting human contact. Check with the client, and/or her or his caregivers, before the session to understand the current condition of the client. Note any specific precautions to the use of touch. Because of the vulnerability of the immune system of those infected with HIV, be sure that you are free of any contagious infections such as a cold or flu.

People with HIV/AIDS do experience a number of adverse effects related to the drugs used to treat the disease. These include:

- **Lipodystrophy:** A disturbance of fat metabolism, lipodystrophy causes uneven distribution of fat in the body. It may involve loss of fat from the face, arms, and legs, and accumulation of fat in other areas, such as the abdomen and back of the neck. When giving massage be sensitive to the clients' feedback regarding touch of these areas.
- **Muscle cramping:** The muscles may be hypertonic. To calm down the cramping and/or to prevent it, use slow, broad, firm pressure. Avoid stretching and overstimulating the muscle tissue.
- **Intestinal distress:** Patients may suffer from diarrhea, and other gastrointestinal symptoms. Use of acupressure points on the small and large intestine meridians can help calm the body, bringing relief.
- **Neuropathy:** This condition affects primarily the nerves of the hands and the feet, resulting in numbness or pain. Keep touch very gentle and respond to the clients' feedback regarding their preferences for pressure and the types of techniques used. If touch is painful, avoid the areas of neuropathy altogether and focus on other areas of the body that give the patient relief.

The greatest benefit of massage for people with HIV/AIDS is relaxation. The fear and stigma that have surrounded this disease place an emotional burden on them which heightens the already difficult challenge of managing the physical symptoms of the disease and the adverse effects of the drugs designed to treat it. Your compassionate attitude and caring use of touch create a safe haven, allowing them to feel at ease in their own bodies.

Osteoarthritis, literally meaning "inflammation of a joint" is a degenerative condition of the joints, characterized by the destruction of articular cartilage, particularly in weight-bearing joints (e.g., the vertebral column, the hip, and the knee joints). There may be overgrowth of bone and the formation of bone spurs. It is usually accompanied by mild to severe pain, and involves progressive loss of function. Usually caused by wear and tear on the joints and consequent irritation and inflammation, it is a common condition in older people.

In providing Comfort Touch, avoid direct contact on the areas of pain and inflammation (eg, the joints themselves). However, broad encompassing contact pressure to surrounding muscles can bring relief. Gentle motion may also be helpful.

Rheumatoid arthritis is a chronic autoimmune disease characterized by inflammatory changes in the joints, particularly those of the hands and the feet. Changes in the synovial membranes and other connective tissues can lead to deformities of the joints and consequent dysfunction and pain. It affects people of all ages.

As with osteoarthritis, avoid direct pressure on areas of pain or acute inflammation. Comfort Touch can bring relief to areas of tension surrounding the affected areas. Work with the patient's feedback to your touch. Simple holding, letting the warmth of your hands penetrate the tissues, can be very soothing. For example, encompass the patient's hands with both of your hands, holding through several complete breaths. You can also incorporate gentle movement of the arm, to help encourage circulation of blood and lymph and to promote greater mobility.

Bursitis and **tendonitis** are inflammations of structures associated with movement in the body. The bursae are small sacs found in the connective tissue in the area of a joint. They are lined with synovial fluid, which acts to reduce friction in areas of movement. Tendons are composed of fibrous connective tissue and attach muscle to bone. Inflammation of these structures is usually the result of injury or overuse. As the individual rests the areas affected by acute inflammation, the swelling and pain can subside, allowing recovery. For many, however, especially the elderly, the condition becomes chronic, neither responding to rest or other treatments. These are painful conditions, affecting life function. For example, chronic inflammation in the trochanteric bursa (in the hip), or tendonitis of the iliotibial band of the upper leg, can severely limit the ability to walk without pain.

As with any inflammation, it is not advisable to apply pressure directly on the area of injury, as this would cause greater pain and/or injury. But it can be useful to use broad, encompassing pressure to the surrounding muscles to help them relax. Also, because of the limitations to movement caused by the pain, massage to facilitate the flow of lymph distal to the area can be useful. For example, use of the *water stroke,* or other techniques of manual lymph drainage can help bring relief to the person suffering from bursitis or tendonitis.

Diseases affecting the nervous system and consequently the function of the muscles range from those which may develop prenatally, such as cerebral palsy, to others, such as Parkinson's disease, that tend to develop later in life. As with other conditions mentioned in this chapter, the benefits of touch can be appreciated by respecting the needs of the individuals you are touching, as well as responding to their feedback. The following is information on some of these conditions. It is by no means a comprehensive listing:

- **Parkinson's disease** is a chronic nervous system disease, characterized by a fine, slowly spreading tremor, muscular weakness and rigidity, and irregularities of the gait. There may be an increased danger of falling either forward or backwards. The speech is often slow and measured. Its onset is more common in people over the age of 50. Massage and the broad compression of Comfort Touch can help to maintain flexibility, and bring relief from pain. Keep in mind that, although speech is difficult, the mental function of people with Parkinson's disease is normal.
- **Multiple sclerosis** is a disease that involves the destruction of the myelin sheaths around both motor and sensory neurons in the central nervous system, resulting in spasticity of muscles, tremors, fatigue, and progressive loss of motor function. Usually it is diagnosed when the individual is between the ages of 20 to 40 years of age. Symptoms of multiple sclerosis can be exacerbating-remitting—meaning that there are episodes of neurologic dysfunction followed by periods of recovery. They may experience pain owing to muscle spasms and hypertonicity. They can benefit from slow, broad deep pressure. Take care not to overstimulate the muscles, as this can cause more spasms. Stress is a common trigger for the onset of symptoms; therefore, the relaxation afforded by massage can be a valuable part of preventative therapy.
- **Amyotrophic lateral sclerosis** (also known as Lou Gehrig's disease) is a progressive condition that destroys motor neurons in the central and peripheral nervous system, leading to the atro-

phy of voluntary muscles. It is usually diagnosed between the ages of 40 to 70 years old. Loss of function can be rapid, leading to death within a year or diagnosis, or patients can plateau and live many years after diagnosis. Loss of autonomic muscle function leads to loss of respiratory function, so many of these people are breathing with the assistance of ventilators. Likewise they lose the ability to swallow, so they may receive nourishment via breathing tubes. But mental function remains high, so that many adapt to communicate using special computerized devices.

- **Cerebral palsy** is a disease stemming from causes occurring before or during birth or in early childhood. Those affected have impaired muscle function, with sometimes random involuntary movements. When touching them do not try to restrain these movements. Rather, move with their movements, as if to dance in partnership with them as they move. Stay very grounded and flexible in your own body for your safety and theirs. Speech may be somewhat impaired, but communication simply requires the willingness to take the time to listen carefully and respond in the moment.

- **Muscular dystrophies** are a group of more that 30 genetic diseases characterized by progressive weakness and degeneration of the skeletal muscles that control movement. Some forms of muscular dystrophy are seen in infancy or childhood, while others may not appear until middle age or later. Functionality and progression of the disease varies widely. Loss of muscle function not only affects the skeletal muscles, but the cardiac muscle and muscles affecting respiratory function.

- **Post-polio syndrome** is a variety of musculoskeletal symptoms and muscular atrophy that create new difficulties with activities of daily living 25 or more years after the original symptoms caused by the viral infection of poliomyelitis. Massage and Comfort Touch can be very helpful in alleviating the pain and fatigue that accompany this syndrome. Listen carefully to the clients' needs and respond to their feedback.

Visual Impairment

Diseases and conditions affecting vision are widespread among people of all ages, but they are most prominent in the elderly, often representing a challenging loss of function. Though Comfort Touch does not directly relieve visual impairments experienced by people, it can help relieve the patterns of compensation to the musculoskeletal system of those affected. For people who have lost significant function of the special sense of sight, Comfort Touch also provides a nurturing pleasurable experience through another avenue of perception—the sense of touch. It helps provide emotional support to those suffering from the trauma of sudden or gradual vision loss.

Conditions of the eyes range from common eyestrain, **myopia** (nearsightedness), and **presbyopia** (age related farsightedness) to diseases which threaten significant loss of vision, such as **cataracts**, **glaucoma**, **macular degeneration** and **retinopathy.** When eyesight is impaired, the individual may suffer from eyestrain or myofascial tension in other parts of the body, as she or he struggles to compensate for the visual impairment. For example, holding the head in awkward positions to "try and see better" can contribute to tension in the head, neck, shoulders and upper back. Decreases in depth perception or sensitivity to light can affect balance, as the individual braces to avoid falling or bumping into objects. Often tension is held in the muscles, even without the conscious awareness of the individual.

The nurturing pressure of Comfort Touch can help to relieve the discomforts of visual impairment through the use of a few simple techniques. *Lift and squeeze* the bellies of the trapezius muscle at the top of the shoulders (see Figure 5-13) to relieve the tension to this general area. *Contact pressure* (see Figure 5-12) and *specific contact circling* (see Figure 5-11) in the bellies of the trapezius muscle can calm the muscle as you provide pressure to the motor points of the muscle. Massage of the upper back using *broad contact pressure* is helpful as shown in Figure 5-5. It is also helpful to apply pressure to specific tonic acupressure points along the occipital ridge—Bladder 10 and Gallbladder 20 as shown in Figure 5-32.

For people with visual impairment, the pressure to these areas of the body should be applied slowly. The contact can be firm according to the preferences of the client. When using any of these techniques, work very closely with the feedback of the client regarding the amount of pressure used and the length of time pressure is held.

Fibromyalgia and Chronic Fatigue Syndrome

Fibromyalgia, also called myofascial pain syndrome, is a condition without specific known cause. People afflicted with these syndromes experience chronic pain and tender points in the muscles, tendons, and other soft tissues of the body. Often they also experience sleep disorders, fatigue, and depression. **Chronic fatigue syndrome** (CFS) is an associated disorder, characterized by extreme fatigue that impairs activities for at least

6 months, in the absence of other known physical or mental diseases. As the quality of life is affected by pain, fatigue and consequent loss of function, these syndromes affect the individual's ability to live to previous levels of activity.

Nurturing massage that adheres to the principles of Comfort Touch can help these individuals to relax more fully. The *broad encompassing compression* of Comfort Touch is especially soothing, and helps to sedate the nervous system. Many people with fibromyalgia report that techniques of conventional massage (ie, gliding and kneading) cause more pain, perhaps because of the highly sensitive nature of their nervous systems.

Many people with these syndromes have searched for cures for their ailments and experience frustration at the lack of effective treatment options.[3] While it is unknown if some past trauma may be associated with the illness, some have been told that their symptoms are all "in their head," and there is no reason they should feel as they do. In other words, they have been invalidated for their own experience. The attitude of respect inherent in Comfort Touch brings emotional as well as physical relief to them. Be very careful to ask the client what she or he needs and respond to this verbal and nonverbal feedback.

Other Conditions

There are many different diseases and conditions affecting one or another of the tissues, organs, or systems of the human body. For example, scleroderma is a condition which can cause a thickening of the skin or other connective tissues in the body. Diseases affecting the kidney, liver, or gastrointestinal tract may cause local pain or systemic pain and/or dysfunction. It is impossible for practitioners of Comfort Touch to be knowledgeable about all known conditions and pathologies, but it is wise to ask either clients or their caregivers for relevant information in order to best serve their needs. Follow Precautions in the Use of Touch. (See Chapter 3.)

Dementia/Alzheimer's Disease

Dementia is the loss of mental function, and can be attributed to various causes, including; **Alzheimer's disease**, **vascular dementia**, **stroke** (also called **cerebral vascular accident** or CVA), and **transient ischemic accident** (TIA). Brain tumors, injury, or other illnesses can also contribute to dementia.

Alzheimer's disease, which is a degenerative disorder of the brain, is the major cause of dementia. It involves shrinkage and death of neural tissue. Most common in people over the age of 65, it causes memory loss, personality changes, disorientation, and eventual loss of physical function leading to death. For their

own safely and the safety of others, most people with Alzheimer's disease must eventually be taken care of in skilled nursing facilities. Increasingly, people with this disease are being cared for in specialized nursing facilities called "memory centers," which are designed to meet the needs of these patients.

Vascular dementia and stroke are other common causes of dementia in the elderly, and result from changes in the cardiovascular system and diminished blood flow to the brain. In severe cases the loss of mental function is progressive. In some cases it is temporary, and the patient is able to recover function with treatment of the underlying circulatory condition.

The loss of cognitive function may be gradual and progressive, as with Alzheimer's disease, or it may be rapid, as with a major stroke. Fear is often a prevalent emotion, especially if someone has awareness of the loss of her or his own mental function.

Touch can provide a comforting connection for people with dementia, no matter the cause. Mental deterioration usually makes verbal communication difficult. In some cases, such as with stroke, the person may be able to formulate clear thoughts, but is unable to communicate clearly, which can be very frustrating. Touch provides a direct link to nonverbal communication.

Because of its steady, predictable contact, Comfort Touch is an especially suitable approach to massage for the person with dementia. This predictability allows the person to feel safe and in control, regardless of their ability to communicate clearly in words. Remember that as a therapist you might never know what clients are actually experiencing or comprehending inside their own minds and bodies. Therefore, it is wise and respectful to give the benefit of the doubt and treat them as if they can hear and understand your words. They will understand the clear intention of your touch. (See Figure 6-9.)

Terminal Illness

Dying is an inevitable aspect of the spectrum of living experience. Personal and societal beliefs and fears about dying influence much of the way people live. The imminent prospect of dying often challenges an individual's beliefs, and can lead to changes in interpersonal relationships with family and friends. Death affects us all, yet it remains one of life's enduring mysteries.

People approaching death have stated that their greatest fear is not death itself, but they fear the pain, or they fear being out of control. Appropriate palliative care, including Comfort Touch, can bring soothing relief into the picture as one faces the pain, fear, and uncertainty surrounding death. To provide palliative care does *not* mean "to assist people to die." Rather, the intention is to help individuals to experience comfort-

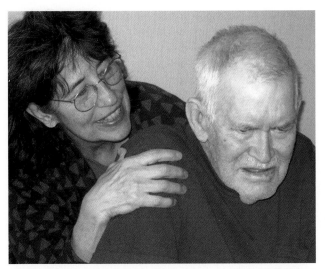

FIGURE 6-9. Connecting with a dementia patient. The caregiver connects with this man using broad, encompassing touch.

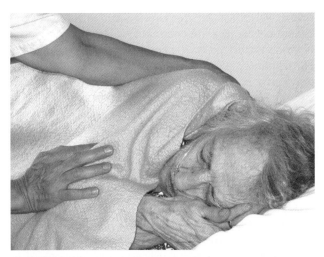

FIGURE 6-10. Encompassing touch. A woman in a long-term care facility relaxes during a session of Comfort Touch.

ing support in an atmosphere of dignity and grace, even until the final moments of life.

For the purposes of insurance coverage for hospice care or the provision of the Medicare hospice benefit, there are established guidelines to predict the course or prognosis of a disease. But the timing of death is not a fixed science. There is tremendous variation in life expectancy among individuals living with chronic/terminal illness. In fact, some people treated with palliative measures recover function, living far beyond their prognosis. For others, death comes quickly, without warning. So the practitioner of Comfort Touch is reminded to be present with the patient, respectful of the opportunity to provide care in the moment.

General Geriatric Decline

The process of aging inevitably leads to death. There are those people for whom there is no specific diagnosis of illness, except for the slow decline in function of all the bodily systems. Referred to as "general geriatric decline," "debility unspecified," or "failure to thrive," the individual may be living at home, in a nursing facility, or in a hospice. Comfort Touch can be a helpful aspect of care, bringing dignity and respect to the aging individual. (See Figure 6-10.)

End Stage of Disease

Terminal illness affects people of all ages and lifestyles, across the spectrum of life circumstances. The leading causes of death are heart disease, cancer, stroke, respiratory illnesses, accidents, diabetes, infectious illnesses, and Alzheimer's disease. Each disease has unique signs and progression of symptoms. When treatment options

are no longer effective in curing or halting the progression of the disease, and when life function is severely affected, the person is said to have a terminal illness. Within the hospice and palliative care model of medicine, efforts shift from the curative mode to that of providing comfort. These palliative measures include pain management, nutrition, personal care of the body, and psychoemotional and spiritual support. The principles and techniques of Comfort Touch are consistent with and complementary to this model.

The following are some of the changes that can be noted in terminal illness:

- **Functionality:** The function of body organs and systems diminishes, affecting changes in mobility, circulation, respiration, digestion, and elimination. There may be changes in vision, hearing, and the ability to speak.
- **Pain:** Levels of pain may necessitate adjustments in the use of pain medication.
- **Emotional expression:** The patient undergoes changes in emotional expression. A person might feel sad, angry, depressed, anxious, agitated, or accepting. *There is no one way that people feel or should feel.* Emotional response can vary by the day or by the hour.
- **Withdrawal:** The patient usually indicates less interest in eating and drinking. She or he might have less interest in social interaction, or wish to limit interaction to a chosen few family and/or friends.

Comfort Touch for the Comatose or Dying Patient

In the practice of Comfort Touch you may have the opportunity to provide touch for someone who is in a

coma. Derived from the Greek word *koma,* meaning "deep sleep," it is the profound state of unconsciousness, characterized by the absence of eye opening, verbal response, and motor response. A coma may be a temporary state (eg, when someone is recovering from surgery or serious injury). A coma may be medically induced, when sedation facilitates the healing process. Or a coma may be part of the trajectory leading to death.

Just because someone cannot speak or move does not mean they do not think or feel or hear. Be especially sensitive to the impact of your presence, your words, and your actions, when you are in the room with someone who appears to be in a coma. *It is best to assume the patient can hear you and others as you speak.* Always include the patient in your awareness.

The following are considerations for providing Comfort Touch to a person who is in a coma or actively dying:

- **Communicate:** Talk as if the person can hear you, introducing yourself and stating your intention to offer Comfort Touch. Ask permission, and take a moment before actually making physical contact. You do not need to hear a verbal response, but your words should convey respect and the intention to comfort, easing the way into the touch itself.
- **Keep the touch simple:** Following the principles of Comfort Touch, let the pace of your touch be particularly slow. *Broad contact pressure* and *holding* are appropriate techniques to use. You may want to sit beside the patient, relaxing in the quiet, still atmosphere.
- **Pay attention to nonverbal feedback:** Notice the patient's nonverbal response. For example, you may observe changes in the pattern of breathing, or note subtle movements in the eyes or other areas of the body.
- **Remember to breathe:** Being in the presence of someone who is close to dying is a very profound experience, and may trigger intense feelings for you. Remember to breathe. Keep grounded. Take a break if you need to.
- **Respect others:** Often other family members or friends will be in the room. Medical personnel may be present. Respect them all, allowing each one to be close to the patient according to their own inclination. In fact, as a Comfort Touch practitioner you can help to encourage others to touch their loved ones. By your example, you set a tone in which all feelings are valid and acceptable. If it feels appropriate, you may provide gentle, comforting touch to the others present.
- **Let go:** This is a time to let go of your own personal attachments. Remember you are there to offer comfort and assurance. Your kindness, along with the loving support of everyone who is with the patient, can help to ease any fear associated with the illness and/or dying process. In their own time, patients will make the transition we know as death.

STORY

Donald

"The long, sweet velvety night in which all pain subsides beckons to me from the far side of dusk."

Donald wrote these words in the autumn of 1990 before his death from acute myeloid leukemia at age 33. Once an enthusiastic outdoorsman and lover of life, he was coming to terms with the fact that the disease process, once in remission after a bone marrow transplant, was again progressing. As a massage therapist with hospice, I had the privilege of getting to know him in the final months of his life.

As his body became gradually weaker, his mind and heart remained clear and strong. During our bodywork sessions he spoke easily to me of his thoughts on death, stating his wish to be conscious and lucid when it happened. He shared his questions, feelings, and concerns about dying. During his remission he had volunteered his time to work with senior citizens, entertaining them with his juggling and playful sense of humor. There he met Kathryn who worked as the activities coordinator. Even as he fell in love with her, he told her, "I'll never be old."

On Saturday, December 15, Donald and Kathryn were joined by family and friends as they declared their undying love in a marriage ceremony. (See Figure 6-11.) Amid the tears, cheers, and laughter, all could feel the preciousness of life, not really believing death could come within the approaching weeks. Donald, vibrant and fully in command the day of the wedding, began to weaken rapidly in the next few days. The pain in his body increased as well as the exhaustion from anemia and bleeding.

On Tuesday he called together his family and friends, taking time to be alone with each one of them. The temperature outside was frigid and snow blanketed the house, but the warmth of heart in this home was tangible. Thursday night as others slept, another friend and I joined Kathryn as she cared for Donald. Throughout the long hours of darkness he lapsed in and out of consciousness. At one point he said, "No one ever told me how to die. I don't know what to do."

Kathryn, though feeling sadness at his approaching departure, steadfastly, courageously, and compassion-

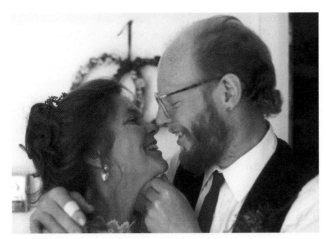

FIGURE 6-11. The wedding day. Living in the moment, Kathryn and Donald celebrated their life together with family and friends.

ately offered encouragement and comfort to him. Softly, she said, "It's okay, Donald. You can just let go."

"That's what's scary," he answered. "You have to let go of everything at once." As the hours progressed through the night, it seemed as though Donald was exploring new territory. His questioning opened up to a different dimension of reality we could only sense but could not see as he could. He said, "It's truly an amazing thing!"

Toward dawn, after a time of deep quiet, he asked, "Is anyone going to go with me on the bus?" He visibly relaxed, peacefully seemed to let go as Kathryn answered, "You have to go alone, but people will be there when you arrive and there will of lots of love where you are going, just as we all love you here. It will be a beautiful trip. Just get on the bus when it comes."

At 6:30 A.M. he spoke his last words, "Kathryn, I love you." Throughout the day he rested comfortably. One or two people were with him all day, simply being present in the silence that Donald emanated and that he valued so much. That night as his breathing changed, we knew death was close. The hospice nurse came. Family and friends gathered to be with Donald in his small bedroom. In our closeness to Donald and each other I could feel the immensity of the emotions surrounding us, and the mystery of death and the magic of life, as we said goodbye to our friend.

At 11:10 P.M. Friday, the evening of the Winter Solstice, he exhaled his last breath. Kathryn, who had offered constant comfort and encouragement throughout the hours and days, now let go of his hand and broke into wailing sobs. "He's gone, he's gone!" The tears flowed freely amidst a chorus of grieving.

"Well, he got the bus!" someone said. Laughter followed, then silence, precious silence.

Many years later, I am still grateful to Donald and his family for the privilege of being with them in their time of transition. There is still so much to learn about life and death and love.

 # Summary

- Inherent to the practice of Comfort Touch is the recognition of the client as a whole human being who can appreciate the value of human connection and compassion.
- Gathering information about the client's condition can ensure the most safe, appropriate, and effective Comfort Touch session possible.
- There might be more variation of symptoms within a group of people who have the same disease than there is among people with different diseases.
- The most appropriate touch sessions for clients are determined by assessing their functionality (physical, mental, emotional), and their level of pain. Always respond to the stated needs and feedback of the client.
- Comfort Touch can bring relief to people needing general emotional support. It can be helpful to people who are suffering from acute trauma or emotional distress, or are suffering from traumatic memories.
- Comfort Touch provides a safe way to massage infants and children. The Comfort Touch practitioner can help to encourage the parent/child relationship through touch.
- Women can enjoy the benefits of Comfort Touch throughout labor, delivery, and the postpartum period.
- Comfort Touch is used successfully in the medical setting for patients suffering from acute illness or injury; before and after surgery; and during the rehabilitation process.
- Comfort Touch is used as part of complementary health care for people suffering from a full range of chronic illnesses and conditions, including: cardiac and pulmonary disease, cancer, diabetes, HIV/AIDS, arthritis, Parkinson's diseases, multiple sclerosis, fibromyalgia, chronic fatigue, and Alzheimer's disease.
- Comfort Touch can provide support throughout the final stages of life.

Review Questions

1. The practitioner of Comfort Touch focuses on the wholeness of the individual. Describe how you would do this when working with someone who has a particular disease.
2. What is the value of studying the pathology of a disease that affects a person who is receiving Comfort Touch?
3. Explain this statement: "There might be more variation of symptoms within a group of people who have the same disease compared with people with different diseases." Give examples.
4. What is meant by the term "functionality?" Give examples. How can the assessment of the client's functionality affect choices made in giving a Comfort Touch session?
5. Why is it important to ask the patient about her or his experience of pain?
6. Explain this statement: "Having something to feel good about is an antidote to pain."
7. Describe how the practitioner of Comfort Touch can be helpful to someone experiencing emotional pain or discomfort.
8. What are the benefits of Comfort Touch for infants and children?
9. Give three considerations for working with patients in a medical setting.
10. List 5 to 10 chronic conditions/illnesses for which Comfort Touch can provide complementary therapy.
11. What is the value of Comfort Touch for people suffering from dementia/Alzheimer's disease?
12. List several changes that can be noted in the end stage of illness. How can the Comfort Touch practitioner provide support through these changes?

References

1. Rose MK. Therapeutic massage and diabetes. *J Massage Ther*. Winter 2002.
2. Rose MK. *Therapeutic Massage and Diabetes. Hypoglycemia: What Massage Therapists and Diabetics Need to Know*. 2006. http://www.comforttouch.com/Hypoglycemia.htm. Accessed August 25, 2008.
3. John J. *A Consensus Manual for the Primary Care and Management of Chronic Fatigue Syndrome*. Trenton, NJ: The Academy of Medicine of New Jersey. March 2002.

Suggested Reading

Beers MH, Berkow R, eds. *The Merck Manual of Geriatrics,* 3rd ed. Whitehouse Station: NJ; 2000.

Greene E, Goodrich-Dunn B. *The Psychology of the Body*. Baltimore: Lippincott Williams & Wilkins; 2004.

MacDonald G. *Medicine Hands: Massage Therapy for People with Cancer*. 2nd Ed. Forres, Scotland: Findhorn Press; 2007.

Werner R. *Massage Therapist's Guide to Pathology*. Baltimore: Lippincott Williams & Wilkins; 2005.

7

Communication and Documentation in the Healthcare System

> I enjoy reading the massage therapists' CARE Notes in the patients' charts. They give me a good picture of what is going on with my patients, and assist me in determining the best care for them.
>
> —Susan, hospice nurse

Communication in the Healthcare System

As therapeutic massage and Comfort Touch take their place as complementary therapies in medical settings, it becomes necessary to communicate with other people in the healthcare system about this service. Clear communication—both verbal and written—establishes professionalism and demonstrates the ability to work with others in providing the best care for patients. Written documentation becomes a part of the medical record of the patient. Client intake information and **CARE Notes**—the system of documentation described in this chapter—can be applied appropriately to the practice of massage and Comfort Touch, whether in a hospital, hospice, skilled nursing facility, homecare, or private practice.

Communication with the Healthcare Team

The ability to communicate the value and benefits of massage therapy and Comfort Touch sets the stage for the practice of these complementary therapies in a medical setting. Proper documentation of completed sessions records the time spent with patients, noting the condition of the patients before massage, the service you provided for them, and their response to the work. This documentation is read by other health professionals who care for the patient, who might include physicians, nurses, nursing assistants, social workers, physical therapists, and other massage therapists. The notes you record become a permanent part of the patient's medical record and, as such, might also be read by insurance claims personnel, or medicare staff.

Communication with the Patient

Prior to the hands-on session, you will introduce yourself to the patient, stating your intention to offer Comfort Touch and/or massage. You might have already seen the client's chart or been informed of the patient's condition, but it is always appropriate to ask the patient if she or he has any special needs at the moment. For example, ask, "How are you? Is there anything in particular needing attention today?" or "Do you have any areas of pain or discomfort you want me to work on?" You can simply ask, "How can I help you today?" Even if the client has limited ability to speak, it is still important to voice these questions and to keep them in your mind as you work.

Remind clients that it is your intention to offer comfort. Say, "Let me know if anything I do is uncomfortable. This should *not* be painful in any way." Throughout the session note their verbal and nonverbal feedback and respond accordingly. See Chapter 3 for further tips on communication with clients. Remember that this aspect of communication creates safety for the client and helps you to determine the most effective treatment. The information gained through direct communication with the patient will contribute to your written documentation after the session is completed.

Guidelines for Written Documentation

Consider the following when charting a massage session:

- **Sign and date all documentation.** The massage therapist's name, along with the date of the session, should always be on the chart.
- **Complete the documentation as soon as possible after the session.** It is easier to write about a session while the experience is fresh. With practice, it should only take a few minutes to accurately complete all the details necessary.
- **Write legibly.** A chart that cannot be read is useless. Print or write legibly. You might want to take quick notes after the session and type them up later. Some facilities use computers directly for all charting.
- **Keep in mind the person(s) who will read the chart.** This documentation is read by other health professionals who care for the patient, who might include physicians, nurses, nursing assistants, social workers, physical therapists, and other massage therapists. Use language that can be understood by others, regardless of their profession. Avoid the use of terms that are vague, intangible, or that might not be understood by others in the medical field. Examples include terms such as "energy work," "chakra healing," and "trigger points."
- **Use precise and correct medical terminology.** It is important to have a good understanding of medical terminology. Understanding the anatomy and physiology of the body should form the basis for education in massage therapy or other health professions. A course of study in medical terminology with an emphasis on the root words that form more complex words is valuable for anyone working in a medical setting. However, the practitioner of Comfort Touch is generally not expected to understand the complete range of terms used in a medical setting. Do not be afraid to ask others what is meant by particular terms. Keep a good medical dictionary available, and refer to it when needed. Avoid vague or imprecise terms. Use correct medical terminology whenever possible. For example, instead of saying: "I massaged her stomach," say "I massaged her abdominal area."
- **Limit the use of abbreviations and symbols.** In order to facilitate clear communication with others reading the chart, it is usually better to avoid the use of abbreviations. While it might save writing time to use standard abbreviations, be aware that there can be various associations among people of different professions or personnel in different medical facilities. The use of abbreviations can help to expedite charting, but be sure that everyone reading the chart knows what the abbreviations mean. For example, a supervisor in one facility was alarmed to find the letters "S.O.B." in the chart of a frail 85-year-old woman, until she realized that the letters meant "shortness of breath."
- **You may use sentence fragments.** It is acceptable to use sentence fragments to save time and space when charting, but make sure they make sense to the reader. The test of an adequate sentence fragment is this: Can the reader easily translate that fragment into a logical sentence that would be consistent with the flow of the information in the chart? For example, "Intermittent pain in right sciatic nerve" can easily be understood as "The client reports intermittent pain in the right sciatic nerve."
- **Be aware of legal ramifications.** Remember that the medical record is also a legal document, which can be used to determine insurance or

Medicaid/Medicare eligibility and reimbursement. Record the *present* condition of the client, the work you do, and the client's response to it. Do not speculate about prior injuries or conditions, or comment on the course of treatment outside of your own practice with the patient.

- **These records are confidential.** Notes are to be read only by authorized people who are involved in the patient's care. They should be kept in a safe place where they are protected from anyone else's view.
- **Keep in mind your scope of practice.** Be consistent with your role as a massage therapist. You can make observations of the client, but you *cannot* diagnose a condition. For example "anxiety" is a medical diagnosis, but you can report what the client says, for instance, "Patient reports feeling worried or 'stressed out.' "
- **Avoid judgment.** Present the facts of what you see, but avoid interpretations. For example, you can say that the patient did not respond to your questions, but avoid saying, "The patient ignored me." Maybe they didn't hear what you asked, or they have difficulty speaking.

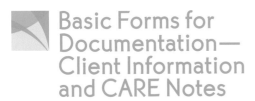

Basic Forms for Documentation— Client Information and CARE Notes

There are two basic forms used in documenting massage therapy and/or a Comfort Touch session: The **Client Information form** records information gathered *before* the initial session with the client. **CARE Notes** document each subsequent session.

Client Information

The initial session with a client begins with completion of a **Client Information** form. This is a document used to record pertinent information about a person receiving massage therapy. It includes the client's name, contact information, medical history, current health condition, and other information relevant to receiving touch therapy. The form is filled out by the massage therapist or Comfort Touch practitioner. The information is obtained by interviewing the client. If the client is unable to answer these questions, the form can be filled out by interviewing one of the client's caretakers. This can be either a family caregiver or another healthcare professional working with the patient.

Depending on the setting in which you work, formats for intake vary widely. If you work in a medical setting or massage clinic, they will provide a standard form, or one will have already been completed for you to see. You might not have access to the patient's chart, but you can ask for information regarding the patient's diagnosis and current medical condition. Ask for any precautions in the use of touch, or recommendations for the use of touch therapy.

A completed Client Information form answers the following questions about the client: "Who are you? How are you? How can I help you?" This information is organized into the three parts of the Client Information form shown in Figure 7-1. Begin by dating the form. Subsequent additions and changes will be dated in the ongoing CARE Notes.

Part 1: Contact Information

Part 1 of the form contains identifying information regarding the client and includes the client's name, gender, and date of birth. It also includes the client's address and phone number(s). Sometimes it is necessary to include contact information of a family caregiver in addition to the client's home address. List the person who referred the client to you.

Part 2: Medical History

Part 2 of the form includes the following information regarding the client:

- **Medical history.** Provide a summary of chronic illnesses, injuries, surgeries, broken bones, etc.
- **Current health conditions or complaints.** Include the client's general health condition and level of mobility and activity. Include special needs, such as the use of oxygen, catheter, requirements for body positioning, and any precautions regarding allergies. Include areas of pain or discomfort.
- **Other medical treatments or therapies.** Include medical treatments, such as chemotherapy, radiation, physical therapy, occupational therapy, speech therapy, and respiratory therapy. Include other alternative or complementary therapies.
- **Medications.** List use of relevant prescriptions or over-the-counter medications.
- **Lifestyle factors.** Include information relating to the client's lifestyle; for example, occupation, physical exercise, hobbies, diet, or smoking habits.

Part 3: Current Reason for Massage

Part 3 of the information form answers the question, "How can I help you?" The reasons for requesting massage and Comfort Touch include relaxation, pain relief, relief of general or specific muscle tension, and

Client Information

PART 1

Name _____ **Date** _____

Date of birth ___/___/___   female _____ male____

Address _____ **Phone** _____

_____ _____

City _____ **State** _____ **Zip** _____

Referred by _____

PART 2

Complete information – Continue on back side of page if necessary.

Medical History *(List chronic illnesses, injuries, surgeries, broken bones, etc.)* _____

_____

_____

_____

_____

_____

Current health conditions or complaints *(Include general health condition, level of mobility or activity, allergies, special needs, areas of pain or discomfort, etc.)* _____

_____

_____

_____

_____

Medical treaments and/or therapies *(Specify medical treatments provided by other health care providers, such as physical therapy, occupational therapy, respiratory therapy, psychotherapy, alternative or complementary therapies.)*

_____

_____

_____

Medications *(List use of prescription and over-the-counter medications)* _____

_____

_____

Lifestyle *(List relevant information regarding physical exercise, actitivies/hobbies, diet and/or smoking habits.)*

_____

_____

PART 3

Reasons for requesting massage therapy *(Relaxation, pain relief, general or specific muscle tension, stress relief, health maintenance, etc.)* _____

_____

_____

FIGURE 7-1. Client Information Form. Complete this form prior to beginning a Comfort Touch session.

health maintenance. Sometimes the needs are psychosocial in nature. For example, the client enjoys the human connection, including verbal and nonverbal communication.

Figure 7-2 gives an example of a completed Client Information form.

CARE Notes

CARE Notes provide a method for documenting massage therapy. This method is appropriate for the full range of massage therapy practice—whether it is used in private practice, or as part of a complementary therapy program in a medical setting. CARE Notes record the *Condition* of the client, the *Action* taken, the *Response* of the client, and *Evaluation* of the session. Consistent with the scope of practice guidelines for massage therapists, it documents relevant information so that necessary precautions are taken in the care of the client, and ensures that appropriate touch techniques are used.

The CARE Note method of charting is compatible with narrative charting practices used by nursing professionals in medical settings. It provides a straightforward, easy, and consistent way to record a client's medical history and present condition, while documenting the massage techniques used and the client's response to the session. This flexible guide allows for comprehensive detail when it is required. It also offers a simple format for concisely recording a massage session when the client's condition is stable over time.

Data from the Client Information form, whether previously filled out by another health professional or the massage therapist at the time of the session, form the basis of the client's medical record. CARE Notes are completed at the end of the first hands-on session and after every subsequent session. They form the ongoing record of the client. The first three elements— *C, A,* and *R*—provide the critical information about a session. They provide a picture of the recipient of the massage, what kind of work was done, and how the individual responded to that work. The fourth element—*E*—is optional, but it allows space to record overall observations, recommendations, or questions that arise from the session.

CARE Notes are completed *after* the hands-on session. Figure 7-3 is an example of a blank CARE Note form. One of these is completed after each session and is entered into the patient chart. Figure 7-4 is an example of a completed CARE Note form. Generally, a massage session is recorded directly onto a form like the one shown. However, in some medical settings the CARE Notes will be summarized and recorded directly into a space provided in the patient chart kept at the nurses' station. It will still include the necessary elements of the *condition of the patient,* your *action taken,* and the *response of the patient.*

Condition of the Client

This section of the chart records the current condition of the client. It should give an accurate picture of the person in the present, and answers the questions, "Who is the client?" and "How is the client now?" This part includes a concise summary of relevant medical information from the client intake form. It will also list current conditions and complaints, areas of discomfort, pain or tension, as well as emotional well-being or state of mind. It records the client's reason for wanting massage, and her or his goals or intentions for the session. If necessary, you can write on the back of the page.

This section can include a notation of physical and/or emotional discomfort or pain *before* the session. For example, you can ask, "On a scale of 1 to 10, with 10 being the worst, how would you describe the level of physical pain or discomfort you are feeling right now?" After the session, you would ask this question again, and record the answer in the Response section of the CARE Note. (See Figures 7-3 and 7-4.)

Action Taken

This section of the chart records what you, the therapist, did during the session. Document the position of the client (i.e., seated in chair, supine, or side-lying in the [type of] bed) as you begin the hands-on treatment. Record the techniques you used and the parts of the body you touched. For example, "Used broad, encompassing contact pressure on the shoulders, arms and hands, with specific contact pressure in the middle trapezius muscle." Note the length of the hands-on session. If you spend time attending to any other needs of the patient, record that also.

The action taken should correspond to the stated needs of the client in the first section (condition of client). It also relates to the work you do in response to the client's feedback during the session. For example, during the session, the client says, "Oh, that feels good on my back, but now my leg hurts." So, then, you would work on the client's legs.

Response of the Client

This section of the chart records the physiological changes noted during and after the session. It includes the verbal feedback of the client, as well as nonverbal responses. You can note changes in breathing, tonicity of muscles, facial expressions, or body positioning. This is also the place to record changes on the pain

Client Information

PART 1

Name *Ellen Carroll*   **Date** *10-15-06*

Date of birth *06 | 15 | 1945*   female _*X*_ male____

Address *1350 Heritage Road*   **Phone** *123-456-7890*

City *Pleasantville*   **State** *WY*   **Zip** *12345*

Referred by *Joan Dewgood, M.D.*

PART 2

Complete information – Continue on back side of page if necessary.

Medical History *(List chronic illnesses, injuries, surgeries, broken bones, etc.)* _____

Type 1 diabetes (dx 1985), asthma, hypothyroid, high cholesterol

tibial fracture (1960), car accident (1992) - whiplash

Current health conditions or complaints *(Include general health condition, level of mobility or activity, allergies, special needs, areas of pain or discomfort, etc.)* _____

moderate activity, shortness of breath with exercise, pain in neck, shoulder

and right upper back, occasional numbness in right hand, allergic to

scented lotion (including essential oils)

Medical treatments and/or therapies *(Specify medical treatments provided by other health care providers, such as physical therapy, occupational therapy, respiratory therapy, psychotherapy, alternative or complementary therapies.)*

physical therapy, yoga therapy and meditation practice

Medications *(List use of prescription and over-the-counter medications)* _____

Levemir insulin, Novolog insulin, pulmicort, synthroid, naproxen (Aleve),

Lovastatin

Lifestyle *(List relevant information regarding physical exercise, activities/hobbies, diet and/or smoking habits.)*

moderate daily walking, whole food diet, non-smoker

PART 3

Reasons for requesting massage therapy *(Relaxation, pain relief, general or specific muscle tension, stress relief, health maintenance, etc.)* _____

relaxation, relief from pain in neck, shoulder and back

FIGURE 7-2. Client Information Form. This is a sample of a completed client information form.

CARE Notes for Massage Therapy

Therapist Name _____   Date _____/_____/_____

Client Name _____   Age _____

Setting _____

Condition of Client

(current medical condition, areas of physical pain or discomfort, special needs, mental and emotional state, etc.)

_____
_____
_____
_____
_____

Before session: _____ physical pain or discomfort (0 = none, 10 = highest level)

_____ emotional pain or discomfort (0 = none, 10 = highest level)

Action taken

(massage techniques used, parts of body touched, position of client, length of session)

_____
_____
_____
_____

Response of Client

(physiological changes noted during and after the session, i.e., breathing and changes in body tissues, nonverbal feedback, verbal feedback, etc.)

_____
_____
_____

After session: _____ physical pain or discomfort (0 = none, 10 = highest level)

_____ emotional pain or discomfort (0 = none, 10 = highest level)

Evaluation

(expectations or plan for next session, recommendations to client, suggestions to other caregivers, etc.)

_____
_____
_____

FIGURE 7-3. CARE Notes. Complete this form after each session.

scale if you are using that detail of the chart. It can also be significant if there are no changes.

Sometimes the response of the client is not what we anticipate or hope it will be. Sometimes what you observe will not seem to match the client's verbal response. For example, she or he will appear to relax, but say, "I don't know what good that did." Conversely, she or he may appear to be tense, but say, "That was wonderful. I feel so relaxed." You might record both,

or simply state the verbal response. Remember that human beings are very individual in their response to touch, and we cannot assume that we know what another person is experiencing.

As a massage therapist you often receive information that no one else on the client's care team has, so it is important to report those observations. For example, you might notice a pressure sore on the client's body, or observe toenails that need to be trimmed. Because

CARE Notes for Massage Therapy

Therapist Name ___Agnes Carroll_____   Date __/ / 06 / 07__

Client Name ___Clara Thompson_____   Age ___75 yo_____

Setting ___Life Medical Center_____

Condition of Client

(current medical condition, areas of physical pain or discomfort, special needs, mental and emotional state, etc.)

Patient has coronary artery disease. Bypass surgery in 1995. Fall in 2000, possibly due to stroke. Weakness in legs, uses wheelchair. Skin is very fragile, bruises easily. Talkative with occasional lapses of memeory. Prior experience of massage is limited, but she is receptive to touch. Wants relief from pain in her neck, shoulder & back.

Before session: ___7___ physical pain or discomfort (0 = none, 10 = highest level)

___5___ emotional pain or discomfort (0 = none, 10 = highest level)

Action taken

(massage techniques used, parts of body touched, position of client, length of session)

Patient in supine position in bed. Used Comfort Touch - broad contact pressure & encompassing - on neck, shoulders, arms & hands. Specific contact pressure on mild trapezius & along occipital ridge. In side-lying position, broad & specific contact pressure to erector muscles of back & sacrum. In supine position, short massage of the feet.

30 minutes

Response of Client

(physiological changes noted during and after the session, i.e., breathing and changes in body tissues, nonverbal feedback, verbal feedback, etc.)

Breathing became slower & deeper. "That feels so good" in response to work on the back. Surprised that foot massage was soothing and not ticklish. Asked when I would come back.

After session: ___4___ physical pain or discomfort (0 = none, 10 = highest level)

___3___ emotional pain or discomfort (0 = none, 10 = highest level)

Evaluation

(expectations or plan for next session, recommendations to client, suggestions to other caregivers, etc.)

Recommend use of small rolled towel under neck to alleviate neck pain. Will follow up with regular sessions 2 times a week.

FIGURE 7-4. CARE Notes. This is an example of a completed CARE Note.

you spend more uninterrupted time with the patient, she or he might tell you something that has not been mentioned to anyone else on the team. If anything you notice warrants immediate attention—for instance, difficulty in breathing, bruising, or excessive pain—make sure that someone else on the healthcare team is notified before you leave.

After the session you can also ask about the level of physical and emotional pain or discomfort of the patient. This feature of the chart is optional, and is used only where appropriate. For example, it can be used with a patient who is hospitalized for surgery or an acute illness. The change in number on the pain scale reveals significant information to the nursing staff. However, if patients are receiving chronic long-term nursing care, their condition is relatively stable, or they are unable to respond to questions, it would be inappropriate to use this scale.

Hints for Practice

Keeping a Personal Journal

Writing in a personal journal can be a valuable part of your learning process, helping you to integrate your experiences into your professional and personal life. Keep a private journal that is separate from the Client Information forms and CARE Notes that are part of the patient's medical record. Respecting the rules of confidentiality, however, do not use patients' names or identifying information in a journal. The focus here is about your <u>own</u> experience. Some elements that can be included in a personal journal might include:

- **Use of techniques:** Record the techniques you used and the effects you observed.
- **Questions and concerns:** Record questions that arise relating to the use of technique, body positioning, communication with the client, or personal issues. Later, you can address these questions or concerns with your supervisor or a trusted mentor.
- **Self-assessment of skill:** Notice your level of confidence in the work you do. Were you able to meet

the needs of the client appropriately and effectively? Did you feel comfortable in your own body as you worked?

- **Evaluation of emotions:** Working with the people you serve can be challenging emotionally as well as physically. How did you feel as you worked? How did you feel after the session? Were there particular emotions that were triggered for you?
- **Integration of personal experience:** Describe your experience in terms of the rewards you gain from doing this work. What is most satisfying to you? What are you learning, and what do you hope to learn?

Here is an example excerpted from the journal of a massage therapist: "When I first started practicing Comfort Touch, it was easy to feel like I wasn't doing a lot. Over time, I am realizing how much I <u>am</u> doing. I see how other people are afraid to touch someone who is sick. They stand back. It reminds me of a time I was very sick in the hospital, and no one touched me. How comforting it would have been to have someone there just to touch me."

Evaluation

This section provides a space to record the overall evaluation of the session. It includes plans or expectations for subsequent sessions, and may include any observation not already recorded. It contains any recommendations made to the client, such as a suggestion to do a simple exercise to alleviate back pain. If the client is being seen by other caregivers, it could include suggestions or relevant information for them regarding the care of the client.

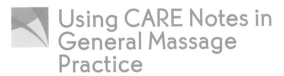

Using CARE Notes in General Massage Practice

The system of charting massage therapy, utilizing the CARE Note format, can be applied to the general practice of hands-on bodywork, whether it is used in a medical setting, a wellness center, a spa, or in private practice. While it is appropriate for documenting Comfort Touch, it can just as easily be used in documenting

other styles of massage, such as Swedish, Integrative, or Neuromuscular Therapy. It is consistent with the scope of practice guidelines for the practice of massage therapy, because it states the client's condition based on a given diagnosis, but does *not* ask the massage therapist to make a medical diagnosis or assessment.

The elements of the CARE Note system fulfill legal requirements for documentation of massage therapy in cases involving insurance reimbursement for personal injury. Just as this system is understandable to healthcare professionals in the medical system, it is understandable to members of the judicial profession. Attorney Linda Herrick underscores the importance of this method of charting, "As an attorney who has worked both as insurance defense counsel and representing plaintiffs who have suffered personal injuries, I believe CARE Notes charting offers concise, understandable information that will be useful to all involved. I would like to see CARE Notes as the standard for massage therapy charting."[1]

CARE Notes are also appropriate for use in an interdisciplinary clinic involving other complementary therapies along with conventional medical approaches. Reliable documentation reflects on the quality of care for the client, promotes continuity of treatment, and facilitates communication among the various healthcare professionals. The act of writing CARE Notes validates the significance of your work.

STORY

Terrible

As a massage therapist I always feel it is a privilege to attend the interdisciplinary team meetings of the hospice where I work. These weekly meetings are attended by the staff members who attend to the needs of the patients—nurses, CNAs, physicians, social workers, chaplains, and, sometimes, homecare volunteers. It is a time to discuss the medical status and needs of the patient, as well as to report on psychosocial issues involving the patient and her or his family.

At one meeting, Sharon, a social worker, talked about one of her patients. She recounted that every week when she sees a particular patient, she asks her, "How are you?" "Terrible," is the woman's reply. Sharon asked the same question with each visit, and heard the same one-word response week after week, "Terrible."

"On my visit this week," Sharon shared with the other team members, "when I asked my usual question, she said, 'Okay.' "

Another team member asked, "So what was different this time?"

Sharon replied, "I checked her chart and noticed that the massage therapist had just been there to give her Comfort Touch."

Summary

- Communication via verbal and written documentation is a necessary skill for practitioners of massage therapy and Comfort Touch within a healthcare system.
- Client Information forms and CARE Notes provide precise and appropriate formats to record client information before and after massage therapy sessions. In a medical setting, they become part of the patient's medical record.
- Guidelines for written documentation include recording the current date, inclusion of the therapist's name, timeliness of completion of charting, legibility, use of understandable and appropriate language, and correct use of medical terminology.
- Charting of massage therapy and Comfort Touch is part of the patient's medical record. Observe professional rules of confidentiality.
- The Client Information form records pertinent information about the person receiving massage. It includes contact information, medical history, and the client's reasons for requesting massage therapy or Comfort Touch.
- CARE Notes provide a precise, appropriate method for documenting massage therapy or Comfort Touch. They record the *Condition* of the client, the *Action* taken, the *Response* of the client, and *Evaluation* of the session.

Review Questions

1. What are the three parts of a Client Information form?
2. Complete an information form for yourself.
3. Complete an information form by interviewing another student.
4. What information is recorded in the "C" section of the CARE Note?
5. What information is recorded in the "A" section of the CARE Note?
6. What information is recorded in the "R" section of the CARE Note?
7. What information is recorded in the "E" section of the CARE Note?
8. After giving a Comfort Touch session to another student, complete a CARE Note chart for that session.

Reference

1. Rose M. The art of the chart: documenting massage therapy with CARE Notes. *Massage and Bodywork Magazine.* 2003; April/May.

Self-Care for the Caregiver

> Listening, we willingly take on some of another's burden for a while, as we might carry a package for a person if we were walking together. At the end of our walk, we give the package back. It is enough that we have been helpful to that person as we have stepped together along our way.
>
> —Maggie Davis

*W*hether it is a parent caring for a child, a friend helping a friend, or a healthcare professional providing services to a client, caregiving forms a significant aspect of human interaction. The instinct and inclination to care for others is the glue that holds a society together. Caregiving is the outer expression of the inner need to connect with others, to belong to something larger than oneself. The concepts and techniques presented in this text are designed to help individuals become more skillful and effective in their roles

as caregivers. This chapter is designed to focus on the health and wellbeing of the ones who are offering care to others.

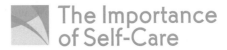

The Importance of Self-Care

The role of caregiver can be a stressful job, involving challenges that are physical, mental, and emotional. The work of hands-on caregiving involves physical exertion, while utilizing the mental capacities involved in making decisions and solving problems. The role of caregiver also requires open-hearted communication with other people and sensitivity to their emotions.

In order to best serve our clients, we must recognize the stresses involved in illness and aging (see Chapter 2). These include physiological processes, psychosocial issues, bereavement, and adaptations to change. By understanding these issues, we are able to support our clients and bring comfort into their lives. By the same token, we need to recognize that these same stresses in our own lives affect our health and our outlook on the world. Through self-reflection, we can keep a balance between the role of caregiving and the need to pay attention to our personal needs.

As sensitive caregivers, we cannot help but be affected by the people we touch who are in pain, whether their pain is physical, mental, or emotional. But awareness of another's pain need not adversely affect our overall health and sense of well-being. To be effective in working with others, we need to pay attention to our own needs, and be deliberate in our program of self-care. We must nourish ourselves through good nutrition and exercise, and maintain a positive attitude. We must also be realistic about the challenges we experience in our own lives, and develop effective ways of dealing with stress and loss.

Wellness Self-Assessment

Given the importance of self-care, it is a useful exercise to take the time to evaluate your own lifestyle. The assessment provided in Figure 8-1 will give you the opportunity to think about the various aspects of your daily living that contribute to your health. Fill out the form, keeping in mind that there are no right or wrong answers.

When you have completed the assessment, notice your overall score. Are you happy with your life as it is? Do you want or need to make changes to create a happier and healthier life for yourself? As you read through this chapter, think about ways in which you can enhance the quality and effectiveness of your self-care.

The Cycle of Health

It is helpful to approach the subject of self-care by looking at the rhythms of the natural world. Attuning to the creative process evident in the cycle of the seasons, we can see patterns that will assist us in bringing a healthy balance of self-care measures into our lives. Figure 8-2 illustrates the four seasons with the free and natural therapies associated with each time of the year. For example, winter is a natural time to rest. It is associated with sleep and stillness. Spring is the season of new growth, and is associated with movement, physical exercise, and activity. Summer is the time of abundance and warmth, naturally associated with nourishing food. It is also a time for connection with others through community activities and travel. Autumn is the time to reap the harvest of the previous seasons, and it is a time to release and let go of whatever is no longer useful. Focusing on the breath—inhalation and exhalation—naturally fits with this season.

Just as we learn by observing the natural cycles of the yearly seasons, so we can learn by respecting the cycle of the day and night. From a place of rest, we move into activity, reaching out for connection and nourishment outside of ourselves. We sleep, we move, we eat, we breathe, we let go, and surrender to the cycle again. Like all living creatures, we live and thrive in natural cycles of activity and inactivity, of nourishment and assimilation, of inspiration and exhalation. We honor the changes within the cycles of the day, the week, the year, and a lifetime.

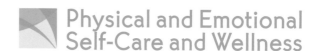

Physical and Emotional Self-Care and Wellness

It is essential to take care of the body's basic needs in order to replenish the physical energy expended in daily living and working. It is also important to care for the emotional, mental, and spiritual aspects of one's self. Following are suggestions for self-care. As you read through, take note of those areas in which you are already conscientious and consistent in your health care. Then notice the areas in which you can bring greater awareness into your life. Make a commitment to explore new ways of nurturing yourself.

Sleep and Rest

Sleep is the primary free and natural therapy for self-care. Think of it as a time to fill the reservoir of energy that has been expended during your waking hours. An adequate amount of quality sleep is required for physical healing and regeneration in the body. Sleep provides a time to let the mind relax into unconsciousness, letting go of the events and cares of the day. Dreaming is an important way to process the activities, thoughts, and feelings of the day.

Generally, 8 hours is thought to be the requirement for adequate sleep. But it is important to respect your own needs, which may be more or less. Your requirements can vary with your activities and the time of the year. It is helpful to establish regular times for sleep, and to create a quiet, dark place that is comfortable and conducive to sleep.

For many people, a short nap or two during the day can supplement nighttime sleeping, allowing the body and mind to relax. Take a few minutes to sit in a comfortable chair with your eyes closed. Daydreaming can help to free the mind and may, indeed, recharge your imagination as you carry on with the day's work.

If you have difficulty falling to sleep at night, try dimming the lights in the evening to help your body and mind switch from an active to a receptive mode for

WELLNESS SELF-ASSESSMENT

Read the following statements and assign a number that most *closely* fits your experience.

4 if you ***agree*** with the statement.

3 if you ***agree somewhat*** with the statement.

2 if you ***disagree somewhat*** with the statement.

1 if you ***disagree*** with the statement.

_____ I am satisfied with the amount and quality of sleep I get each day.

_____ I am satisfied with the amount of exercise I get on a weekly basis.

_____ I typically have enough energy to do what I want to do in a given day.

_____ My diet consists primarily of whole, natural foods.

_____ I feel confident that my diet meets all of my nutritional needs.

_____ I drink an adequate amount of pure water each day.

_____ I drink alcoholic beverages only in moderation.

_____ I am aware that I usually breathe fully and easily.

_____ I abstain from smoking.

_____ I am satisfied with my weight (within 5 lbs).

_____ I am satisfied with my overall physical appearance.

_____ I am satisfied with my present occupation (may include career and/or volunteer work).

_____ I am satisfied with the environment in which I work (lighting, ventilation, ergonomics, aesthetic appeal).

_____ I enjoy the community in which I live.

_____ I enjoy my home life.

_____ I have satisfying relationships with my family and friends.

_____ I take time regularly to enjoy hobbies and/or other creative pastimes.

_____ I have regular medical and dental checkups.

_____ I always fasten my seatbelt when in a motor vehicle.

_____ All things considered, I feel I am living life as fully as I can.

SELF-ASSESSMENT: Add the numbers.

If your total is over 70: Consider yourself healthy. Keep it up!

If your total is over 50: There's room for improvement. Decide where you want to start.

If your total is under 50: It is time to start taking care of yourself!

FIGURE 8-1. Wellness Self-Assessment. Complete this form as a way to evaluate factors relating to your own self-care and wellness.

sleep. Relaxing exercises or a hot bath before bedtime can help you to fall asleep and enhance the quality of your sleep. Hot herbal teas such as chamomile, catnip, or skullcap are soothing and relaxing. (Avoid valerian, as it is stimulating for many people.) Avoid activities that may stimulate you to think too much, such as late-night phone conversations or checking e-mail.

Movement and Exercise

The human body is designed to move. From the simple exertion of daily activities to the focused movement of rigorous exercise, the cells of the body are nourished as oxygen and metabolites are carried through the circulating blood and lymph. The nervous

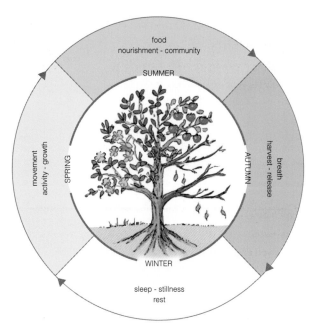

food
nourishment - community

SUMMER

movement
activity - growth

SPRING

breath
harvest - release

AUTUMN

WINTER

sleep - stillness
rest

FIGURE 8-2. Self-care through the seasons. This diagram correlates the various aspects of a healthy lifestyle with the cycle of the seasons. Winter is the time for rest and sleep; spring is the time for movement and growth; summer is the time for food and nourishment; and autumn is the time to focus on the breath and letting go. This cycle of free and natural therapies also correlates with the different times of the day, the week, a year, or a lifetime.

system is stimulated, and changes in body chemistry affect one's mood. Movement is an everyday part of self-care—whether through attention to body patterning during work, or use of therapeutic and recreational exercise.

Body Patterning in Work

Because the occupation of hands-on caregiving involves physical exertion, it is important that practitioners observe the most effective principles of bio-mechanics (see Chapter 3, "Body Patterning for the Practitioner"). As you work, pay attention to your patterns of movement. Take the time that is necessary to find safe and comfortable ways to use your body as you adapt to the needs of the client.

Therapeutic Exercise

There are many different forms of exercise that promote improved circulation in the body and can be used to help strengthen and tone the muscles (e.g., walking, running, swimming, and bicycling). Other types of exercise help to stretch and/or relax muscles, tendons, and ligaments (e.g., yoga, Tai Chi, Qigong, Pilates). Practicing a balance of these exercises helps to optimize

general health, while allowing a break for the stresses of daily life.

The following are several simple exercises that are particularly useful for hands-on caregivers. They all help to stretch, extend, and relax the back, shoulders, and arms, thereby countering the overuse syndromes common to massage therapists. See Figures 8-3 through 8-8.

Recreational Exercise

Many forms of exercise can be considered both therapeutic and recreational. Examples include bicycling, canoeing, dancing, skiing, and competitive sports. You

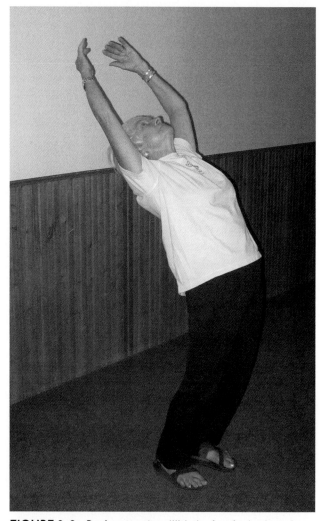

FIGURE 8-3. Back extension. With the feet firmly planted on the ground, lift the arms overhead, reaching upward, elongating the spine. Looking upward, let the body extend backward into an arch. The shoulders should be relaxed down from the ears. Feel the connection of the arms down through the latissimus dorsi muscles of the arms and back. The muscles of the abdomen, low back, and gluteal muscles are contracted to support the extended back. Extend only as far as comfortable, avoiding strain.

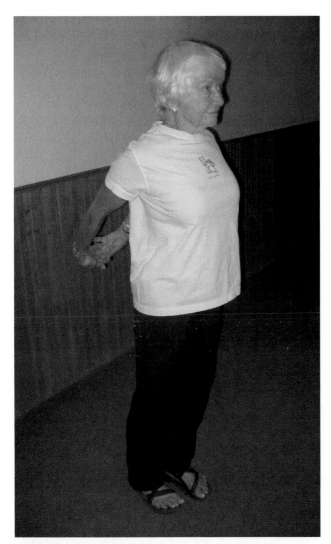

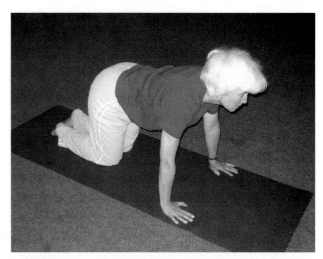

FIGURE 8-5. Cat stretch—starting position. Kneel on all fours, with the hands beneath the shoulders and the knees beneath the hips. Extend the spine and look forward.

body. Good sources of protein are lean meat, poultry, fish, eggs, milk, nuts, seeds, and beans.
- **Fat.** Made up of essential fatty acids, dietary fat is necessary to the assimilation of fat-soluble vitamins, the production of hormones in the body, lubrication of tissues in the body, and to healthy skin and hair. Healthy fats include olive oil, coconut oil, nut butters, and organic butter.
- **Carbohydrates.** Abundant in many foods, carbohydrates provide fuel for the body's cells, and are supplied by a large variety of fruits, vegetables, grains, and beans. Milk and yogurt contain protein, fat, and carbohydrates.

FIGURE 8-4. Chest expansion. Bring the arms behind the back, intertwining the fingers of the hands. Inhaling deeply, feel the expansion of the ribcage, the stretch of the pectoralis muscles, and the retraction of the rhomboids. Focus on letting the muscles of the face and neck remain relaxed.

can enjoy the physiological benefits of these activities, while also enjoying the social connection with other people and the healing benefits of being outside in nature that they afford.

Nutrition

Good nutrition forms an essential aspect of self-care. A diet consisting of whole, natural foods, with proper balance of **macronutrients,** nourishes the individual physically, mentally, and emotionally. These macronutrients include:

- **Protein.** Made up of amino acids, protein is essential to the building and repair of tissues in the

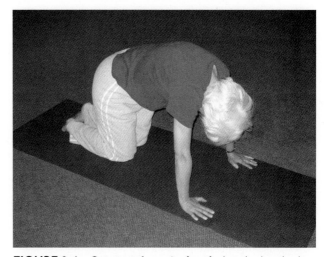

FIGURE 8-6. Cat stretch—spinal arch. Let the head relax downward, while lifting the spine into an arch. Hold this position through an inhalation and exhalation, then return to the extended spine. Slowly, alternate the two positions several times.

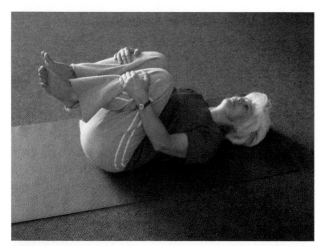

FIGURE 8-7. Knee hug. Let the back relax completely, as you bring your knees to your chest, holding them with your hands. Focus on letting the entire surface of your back make contact with and sink into the floor. Rock gently from side to side, allowing the muscles of the back to be massaged through contact with the floor.

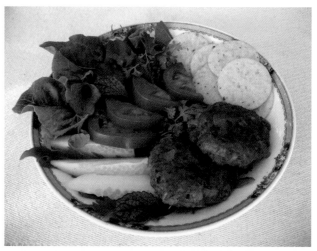

FIGURE 8-9. Nutrient-dense food. This combination of salad greens and vegetables with turkey burgers and rice crackers is an example of an easy-to-prepare nutrient-dense meal. Appealing in appearance, taste, and texture, it has a balance of macronutrients and micronutrients.

Micronutrients are substances found in food that are essential to good health. They include a myriad of vitamins and minerals. It is necessary to eat a variety of foods in recommended quantities to ensure adequate nutrition. A key concept to consider in making healthy food choices is **nutrient density.** This term refers to foods that are high in nutrient content relative to the number of calories they contain. See Figure 8-9.

While the diet should consist primarily of nutrient-dense foods, avoid eating those that contain too many **empty calories.** These are foods such as refined sugar

and flour, which provide calories—and thus can contribute to weight gain—but do not contain appreciable nutrient content. Other substances found in foods may be considered anti-nutrients, because they have potential harmful effects. For example, hydrogenated fats (transfats), food additives, and preservatives should be avoided.

Here are some other points to remember:

- **Read food labels.** Familiarize yourself with the nutritional value of packaged foods by reading the ingredients and nutrient contents listed on the labels.
- **Drink nourishing beverages.** Drink plenty of pure water every day. Green tea, herbal teas, and fruit juices are healthy choices for beverages.
- **Prepare food carefully.** Cooking and preparation of food should optimize its nutrient content, texture, and appearance.
- **Plan ahead.** It is possible to eat well if you plan ahead. For example, cook extra food for dinner, to either eat for a later lunch or save in the freezer.
- **Enjoy food with others.** Sharing healthy food with others adds to the satisfaction gained from eating.
- **Celebrate with food.** It's okay to be flexible with your diet to allow yourself to celebrate special occasions with special foods.

Breathing and Relaxation

Breathing is an automatic function of being alive in a human body. We breathe, whether we think about it or not. By working consciously with our breath, we

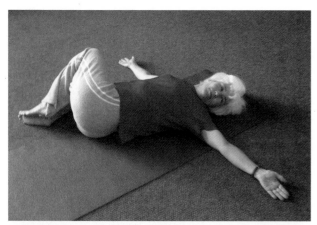

FIGURE 8-8. Knee down twist. Begin in the knee hug position. Extend the arms out to the sides, palms facing upward. Looking in one direction, slowly lower the knees to the opposite direction. Focus on letting the back, neck, shoulders, and arms relax in this position. Slowly, lift the knees to the center, then lower to the other side, as the head turns in the opposite direction.

can improve the effectiveness of our breathing patterns to both energize and relax our bodies. The following are several breathing and relaxation exercises. As you practice each one, notice how it affects your energy level and mental/emotional state of being. It only takes a few minutes a day to experiment with any of these exercises.

Conscious Breathing

One of the easiest and most effective ways to deal with stress is to become conscious of your own breathing. Slow, deep breathing helps you to cope with physical and emotional distress in the moment, and to create a healthy habit for everyday living. Conscious breathing is a way of *letting go of* (exhaling) your own discomfort—physical, emotional, or mental—and it is a way of *taking in* (inhaling) the life force necessary to nourish your body and enhance your sense of well-being.

To become aware of your breath:

1. Place a hand on your abdomen, just below the navel, and let your belly expand as you inhale to allow for a deep and full breath.
2. Let the abdomen flatten as you relax and exhale.
3. Repeat several times.

Practice this exercise anywhere, and any time of the day. Even a breath or two taken consciously can shift your awareness and allow a change of perspective.

Breathing With the Pulse

Sit comfortably in a chair or on a cushion on the floor, and close your eyes.

1. Place the fingers of one hand along the radial pulse points of the other hand (at the wrist below the base of the thumb).
2. Inhale to the count of 4 pulse beats, and then exhale to the count of 4 pulse beats.
3. Continue to inhale and exhale with your pulse, and enjoy the relaxation that comes with tuning into your body this way.

During this exercise, you can continue to hold the pulse points, or let go and continue to relax and notice your breathing. The pulse may change or slow down in this process. Be aware that the pulse can be variable, weak, or pounding. Don't be concerned about the character of the pulse; simply do the exercise as given, and notice the pulse without judging or analyzing it.

Even a few minutes of this practice can calm your body and mind. This exercise is particularly helpful in allowing you to get in touch with what your body needs at the moment.

Letting Go

This exercise provides a simple introduction to the benefits of meditation. It can be useful with as little as 5 to 10 minutes of practice. Gradually increase the time to 20 to 30 minutes.

1. Sit comfortably, close your eyes, and begin to notice your breath. Don't try to change your breathing or do anything in particular.
2. Simply continue to breathe, letting go of each exhalation.
3. As you become aware of bodily sensations, feelings, or emotions, observe them and let them go, as if you were watching clouds pass by.
4. As thoughts come into awareness, observe them and let them go. Don't try to push them away; simply let them go.

This practice helps you to feel at ease with the world around you without being attached to it and therefore controlled by it.

Grounding Visualization

Regular practice of this exercise will enhance the quality of your body patterning when practicing hands-on caregiving or other daily activities.

1. Sit comfortably in a chair and close your eyes. Feel the weight of your body as it contacts the chair.
2. Bring your awareness to your sacrum at the base of your spine. Picture each vertebrae of the spinal column, one stacked upon the other. Notice that the head rests comfortably on top of the neck and back.
3. From the base of your spine, imagine a cord of light that goes all the way into the center of the earth. This is your connection to the earth, your "grounding cord" into the earth.
4. Let anything you wish to let go of—tension, pain, physical or emotional discomfort—be released through this grounding cord into the earth. Trust that the earth can take whatever is released and transform it into neutral energy.
5. Now bring your awareness to your feet and feel the energy of the earth come into your body through the soles of your feet.
6. Follow this flow of earth energy as it moves up through your legs and into the whole torso of your body. Let it fill your neck, face, and head. Let it flow into your arms and hands.
7. Imagine the life force energy as it nourishes your whole body. You can visualize it as a color of light or a stream of water. It can be warm or cool, depending on your preference.

Hints for Practice

Hand Washing: Self-Care Awareness

Washing your hands before and after a session of giving touch is a practical necessity, but it also can be used as an opportunity for self-care on more than one level. Before a session, it can be taken as a time to focus your intention on the work you are about to do. For example, as I wash my hands, I think to myself, "Now I let go of distractions, worries, and concerns, so that I can be fully present while I am with this person for whom I am caring." After the session, as I wash my hands, I enjoy the warmth of the water relaxing my hands and think to myself, "Now I let go of this person's energy, with gratitude for what I have shared and learned in this time. I am now free to move on with my day."

Begin by imagining this process. With practice you will come to know when you are "grounded," and you will feel the peacefulness and confidence that come with this awareness.

Further Suggestions for Self-Care

With respect to your own needs and personality, find an appropriate balance between time for yourself and time for others. Learn to acknowledge your feelings honestly, and find healthy avenues for emotional expression. Remember the importance of humor, and relish the joyous moments in life. Beyond the basics of everyday self-care, there are many ways to nurture yourself.

- **Hobbies.** Whether enjoyed alone or shared in the company of friends, many activities help to alleviate stress. These include watching movies, reading, playing games, or spending time enjoying a favorite craft. Hobbies provide a distraction from the cares and challenges of work. They also provide an avenue for creative expression. See Figure 8-10.
- **Music.** Listening to music can be soothing and energizing. Singing or playing a musical instrument is an avenue for creative expression, and can provide a healthy outlet for emotional energy.
- **Journaling.** Writing or drawing in a personal journal provides another way to express and process thoughts and feelings. Let the words or images flow without editing or self-judgment. The process of letting something flow onto paper without judgment is more important than the content or the finished product.
- **Massage.** Enjoy the physiological and psychological benefits of bodywork for yourself. Not only is this important for your own health and well-being, but as you receive massage, you are reminded of the importance of the caring touch you provide for others.
- **Hydrotherapy/baths.** Take advantage of the healing qualities of water. Take a hot bath with Epsom salts to relax tired muscles. Other hydrotherapy options include whirlpool baths, saunas, steam baths, and foot soaks. Add scented herbs or oils, if these are soothing to you.
- **Flowers/objects of beauty.** Surround yourself with plants, flowers, and/or objects of beauty. Let yourself be nurtured by the colors and textures of natural or artistic objects.
- **Simple rituals.** For many people, simple rituals are an important part of self-care. They can help caregivers to cope with the experiences of death and loss. Rituals can be very personal or they can be shared with others. Here is an example: Lighting a candle is a way of honoring the spirit of someone who has died. Sit for a few minutes and allow yourself to appreciate all that you have learned by your interaction with that person.

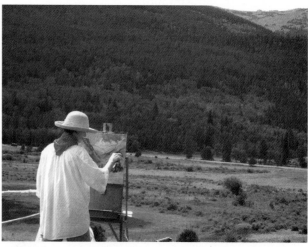

FIGURE 8-10. Hobbies. Enjoy a pastime that provides an avenue for creative expression.

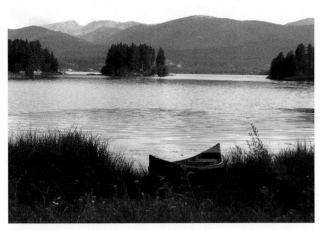

FIGURE 8-11. Time in nature. Enjoy the soothing beauty of the natural world; allow yourself to relax and revitalize.

- **Time in nature.** Spending time in nature is restful and rejuvenating, whether it involves going for a hike, gardening, or resting in the shade of a tree. Enjoy the elements of water, earth, sun and fresh air. Tuning into the natural world reminds you of the cyclical nature of life, and that life persists throughout the changing seasons. You can draw on these soothing images of nature to help relax when you find yourself in a more challenging or stressful environment. See Figure 8-11.

Boundary Issues and Self-Care

Boundaries define the containers within which we live, work, create, and relate to others. They clarify our professional and personal roles. While they may limit certain interactions, they also allow us to focus our attention where it is most needed and appropriate. In the helping professions, regard for appropriate boundaries is considered an ethical issue. Rules of ethics are meant to protect the patient/client. But boundaries are also important to self-care. They protect the caregiver by providing guidelines for making wise decisions in the process of caring for others.

- **Scope of Practice.** Observe the legal scope of practice of your profession. Unless you are a physician (or in most states a nurse practitioner or physician's assistant), you may not diagnose medical conditions, or prescribe medical treatments. Different medical settings and organizations will specify which practices suit your training. For example, in a hospital setting, a massage therapist may require the assistance of nursing staff to transfer or reposition a patient.

- **Roles and agreements.** Keep your interactions within the role for which you are trained and assigned. Keep these questions in mind, "What have I agreed to do in this setting or situation?" "What role do I play?" If a patient makes a request of you that seems inappropriate to your training or role, you can say refuse by saying, "No, I am not qualified or allowed to do that." For example, it would be inappropriate to give medicine to a patient if that is not your assigned role. In another example, a client might request that you use a massage technique that you think could cause tissue damage or pain. If you are in doubt about the appropriateness of a client's request, you can respond by saying, "I will need to ask my supervisor about that."

- **Intimacy.** Hands-on caregiving involves varying degrees of intimacy. Giving and receiving touch *is* enjoyable, soothing, and pleasing to the senses. For either party—the caregiver or the client—feelings of sensuality, sexuality, longing, or attraction can be present, often triggering other feelings of fear, guilt, or confusion. This is a complex issue, but it is important to acknowledge your own feelings and honor the process that brings this issue to the conscious mind. By being honest with yourself, you can deal with these feelings in yourself and others in a way that is clear, respectful, and ultimately freeing. You do not need to be a victim of your own feelings or those of others. Keep in mind your roles and agreements and your ability to say "No," whether to the client's energy and desires or to your own.

Professional Support

With time and attention to self-care, we create the balance necessary to ensure our personal health and well-being. As healthcare professionals, it is also wise to look for ways to nurture ourselves professionally, through peer support and ongoing education.

Peer Support

It is helpful to talk to other professional caregivers who can empathize with the challenges inherent in the work you do. With all due respect for confidentiality, you can discuss questions and concerns relating to your work. Peers also learn from each other and benefit by sharing their successes. If you work within an organization, team meetings can provide useful opportunities to talk about your work and share insights and helpful suggestions.

Mentoring/Supervision

A trusted teacher or supervisor can be a source of encouragement and advice as you pursue your career as a caregiver. Look to someone who serves as an inspiring example of a healthy caregiver. Share your questions and concerns. Offer to assist an experienced teacher or practice your Comfort Touch skills on her or him in exchange for their feedback.

Continuing Education

Ongoing education is a way to keep yourself updated with information that is helpful to you and your clients. Your profession may require continuing education as part of licensing or certification renewal. It is also a way to extend your network of peers, and foster greater opportunities to enhance the practice of your profession.

STORY

A Time to Receive

I opened the front door just after the doorbell rang and saw the box of flowers delivered on my front step. Who are these from? It isn't even my birthday. I opened the box, and put the assortment of budding lilies into the vase provided before reading the card. "Best wishes for a speedy recovery." The flowers were from a group of coworkers.

It had been a few days since I underwent surgery to halt the progression of glaucoma. That morning at the follow-up visit, the doctor seemed well pleased as he checked the pressure in my eye. "Continue to take it easy," he said. "No lifting or bending over for a few more weeks." I felt relief and gratitude for the quality of medical care I was receiving, as well as all the support from family and friends.

The day before the surgery, a group of my women friends came to visit. They asked me to lie down in the center of the circle they formed. Though I was happy to see them, I was reluctant to be the focus of attention. "Mary, it's time for you to receive," they asserted. They acknowledged the times I've been there for them and others in both my personal and professional life. So I lay down on a soft blanket, supported by pillows.

They listened as I shared my hopes and fears regarding the pending surgery. As each woman offered her best wishes for me, she placed a special colored bead on an elastic string. Then they tied this strand of beads on my ankle, a reminder of their care and concern.

These beautiful beads, along with gifts of food, flowers, kind words, and massage accompanied me through the process. As someone who is most accustomed to caring for others, I realized the need to let go of that role as I rested and recovered from surgery. The circlet of beads reminds me that it is an important part of self-care to know when it is time to receive.

Summary

- Caregiving involves many stresses and challenges that are physical, mental, and emotional. It is important that the caregiver pay attention to her or his own needs for care, in order to maintain good health.
- The Wellness Self-Assessment provides a way to evaluate one's own lifestyle. It gives the opportunity to become aware of a wide range of factors that affect your overall health and sense of well-being.
- The Cycle of Health is a visual way to recognize the cyclical nature of self-care, recognizing our basic needs for rest, movement, nutrition, and healthy breathing.
- Regular, quality sleep and rest are essential to good health.
- Movement is an everyday part of self-care—through attention to body patterning during work, and the use of therapeutic and recreational exercise.
- Good nutrition includes a diet consisting of whole natural foods with a balance of macronutrients and micronutrients. A healthy diet includes foods that have a high nutrient density, and a minimal amount of empty calories.
- By working consciously with our breath, we can improve the effectiveness of our breathing patterns to both energize and relax our bodies.
- Beyond the basics of everyday self-care, other activities nurture the body, mind, and spirit. These include participation in hobbies, enjoyment of music, journaling, receiving massage or hydrotherapy, appreciation of beauty, practicing meaningful rituals, and enjoying time in nature.
- Boundaries clarify professional and personal roles. Rules of ethics protect both the client and the caregiver. They are important to the self-care of the care-

giver, because they provide guidelines for making wise decisions in the process of caring for others.
* Professional support can nurture you personally and professionally through peer support, mentoring, and continuing education.

 # Review Questions

1. List the three biggest challenges you face as a caregiver, whether they are physical, mental, or emotional.
2. Complete the Wellness Self-Assessment.
3. Which three aspects of your self-care are the most satisfactory?
4. Which three aspects of your self-care are the least satisfactory?
5. Which two or three aspects of your self-care are you ready to make a commitment for change?
6. Practice the set of therapeutic exercises (Figures 8-3 to 8-8) and describe how you feel their benefit in your body. (You can practice these every day for a week and notice the effect on your body.)
7. Give three examples of nutrient-dense foods. Give three examples of foods with empty calories.
8. Practice at least one of the four breathing and relaxation exercises and describe how it makes you feel. (Practice at least one each day for a week and notice the effect on your body.)
9. Give an example of a situation involving an ethical boundary issue and describe how you would handle it.
10. Describe how peer support and continuing education can support you as a healthcare professional.

Suggested Reading

Davis MS. *Caring in Remembered Ways*. Blue Hill, ME: Heartsong Books; 1999.

Feinberg School of Medicine. Caregivers urged to take care of themselves [on the Internet]. November 2007. http://www.medschool.northwestern.edu/newsworthy/2007B-November/caregivers.html. Accessed November 25, 2007.

Foster MA. *Somatic Patterning: How to Improve Posture and Movement and Ease Pain*. Longmont, CO: EMS Press; 2007.

Hass E. *Staying Healthy with the Seasons*. Berkeley, CA: Celestial Arts; 2003.

Keidel GC. Burnout and compassion fatigue among hospice caregivers. *American Journal of Hospice and Palliative Medicine*. 2002;19:200–205.

McIntosh N. *The Educated Heart: Professional Boundaries for Massage Therapists, Bodyworkers, and Movement Teachers*. 2nd ed. Baltimore: Lippincott Williams & Wilkins, 2005.

Developing a Comfort Touch Program: Administrative Guidelines

> The principles of Comfort Touch—slow, comforting, respectful—can serve as a mantra for any busy health professional. This work has proven to be practical and engaging. It possesses a simple beauty since it articulates not just a method, but a way of being with those in physical, emotional, or spiritual distress.
>
> **—Patrick Davis**

*A*s discussed throughout this text, the intentions and techniques inherent in the practice of Comfort Touch make it ideally suited for a broad range of clientele in a wide variety of settings. This chapter provides information to assist administrators of healthcare facilities who are interested in incorporating Comfort Touch into their programs of care. Likewise, it will give the individual practitioners of Comfort Touch guidelines for approaching facilities into which they wish to offer their skills.

 ## Administrative Overview

As a complementary therapy, Comfort Touch can safely and easily be incorporated in healthcare settings as an adjunct to conventional medicine and nursing care. It can be administered in a number of different ways depending on the management focus of the particular facility in which it is practiced.

Settings for Comfort Touch

The possibilities for the implementation of Comfort Touch programs are numerous. The mission statements of many healthcare organizations include a commitment to the inclusion of complementary therapies with an appreciation for the value of human touch in caregiving. Hospitals, hospices, assisted-living, and skilled-nursing facilities are welcoming the skills of people trained in massage therapy to provide safe, appropriate, and nurturing touch for their patients and residents (Figures 9-1 through 9-4).

Administration of Comfort Touch Programs

Programs of Comfort Touch in healthcare settings can be managed in a number of different ways depending on the populations being served, the settings of the facilities, and the administrative structure of the organization.

Client/Patient Population and Focus of Care

Consider the population being served by a particular healthcare organization or facility. For example, a community hospital may serve a general population, including those in emergency care, and perinatal, surgical, and medical patients. A hospice generally serves the needs of the chronically and terminally ill. Other facilities focus on a variety of specialized needs (eg, rehabilitation, cancer care, or skilled nursing).

Understanding the focus of care is helpful when looking at the specific needs of the people being served. While the primary intention of Comfort Touch is always to comfort the client, it is useful for administrators and practitioners to orient their programs to complement other medical treatments and therapies being offered

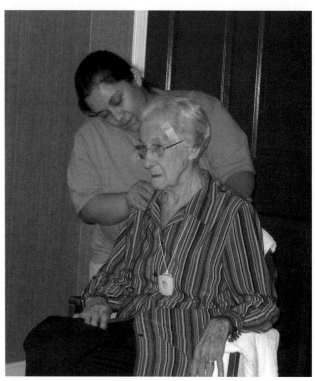

FIGURE 9-2. Comfort Touch in an assisted-living home. A nursing assistant comforts a resident of an assisted living facility.

by the facility. For example, Comfort Touch can provide a welcome balance for the patient who is undergoing rehabilitation after illness or injury, by affording relaxation and reduction of pain. Similarly, Comfort Touch can help to allay the loneliness and isolation, created by the processes of illness and aging, of an elderly patient in a hospice or homecare setting.

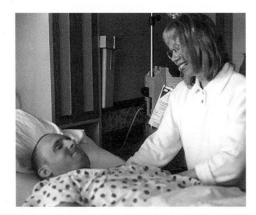

FIGURE 9-1. Comfort Touch in a hospital. Karen Gibson, a nurse massage therapist and pioneer in the hospital-based massage therapy movement, offers the benefits of touch to a patient in a cancer care center of a hospital.

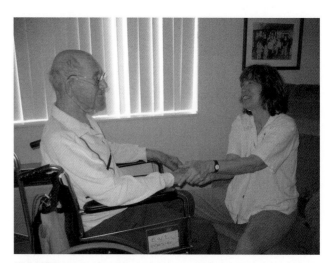

FIGURE 9-3. Comfort Touch in a skilled-nursing facility. A resident of a skilled-nursing facility enjoys the benefits of touch provided by a certified massage therapist.

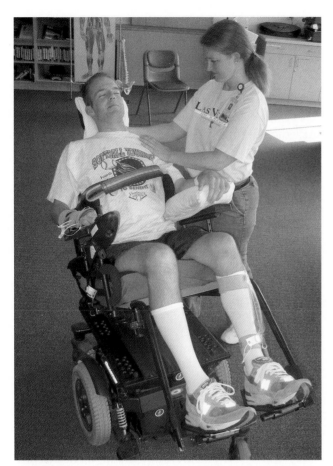

FIGURE 9-4. Comfort Touch in a rehabilitation hospital. A registered nurse provides Comfort Touch to a patient in a rehabilitation hospital. The patient is able to relax in a semi-reclined position in the power tilt chair.

Physical Setting of the Healthcare Organization

The physical settings that house healthcare vary tremendously in structure, size, and in the environments in which they exist. The larger the organization, the more complex is its administrative structure. In a larger organization, a program of touch therapy may be initiated in one area of care, later to expand into other departments. Many medical centers are part of larger, multifacility organizations.

Home healthcare services can be an adjunct to inpatient medical centers, or they can be primary care programs that specialize in the care of patients in their own homes. Touch therapy programs administered through home care agencies require particular care in the hiring of touch practitioners, as direct supervision is more difficult to provide. The majority of hospice organizations are licensed home care agencies, providing direct services to patients in their homes. Home care agencies have central administrative offices with provision for clinical staff meetings and trainings.

Administrative Structure

Healthcare organizations can be either for-profit or non-profit businesses. While either structure can provide excellent quality of care, the chain of accountability may vary, as well as the interface with community activities, such as fundraising efforts to support facilities or services.

Administration of a touch therapy program can be provided in various ways, depending on the size and existing management of the healthcare organization. The structure of the organization will determine how referrals are made for Comfort Touch. Most often, requests for services come from clinical staff working with a patient (eg, nursing personnel or social workers). Some programs require specific permission of the physician involved with the patient. Others give tacit medical approval, owing to the fact that Comfort Touch is a safe and appropriate intervention in a medical setting when performed by trained practitioners of this modality.

Any of the following personnel may be involved in a program.

- **Director of clinical services:** Typically, the director of clinical services is a registered nurse who supervises all personnel who provide services directly to patients. This group would include nurses, nursing assistants, social workers, physical therapists, and occupational therapists. In some facilities, this also includes services provided by chaplains and providers of complementary therapies, such as massage therapy, music therapy, and art therapy. The director of clinical services works closely with the physician in charge of medical decisions (the medical director).
- **Wellness coordinator:** The wellness coordinator is charged with providing ongoing programs in personal fitness, including education in therapeutic exercise and nutrition. Programs vary widely, depending on the interests and needs of the community being served and the resources available. The wellness coordinator might be the one who oversees referrals for massage. In addition to serving the needs of the residents, she or he might coordinate activities designed to promote employee wellness.
- **Complementary care coordinator:** As complementary therapies, including massage, are being used more in medical facilities, a complementary therapies coordinator might hold the responsibility for screening, scheduling, and supervising these therapies. Complementary care can also be a part of employee wellness programs.
- **Activities coordinator:** Most residential facilities, including independent-living retirement homes, assisted-living and skilled-nursing facili-

ties, have an activities program to provide social and educational opportunities for the residents. These can include a wide range of activities designed to provide for the physical, emotional, and mental well-being of the individual. Activities can involve participation in arts, crafts, music, excursions, lectures, and other social events. The activities coordinator might want to include an introduction to Comfort Touch as an activity for residents. For example, a skilled practitioner of Comfort Touch can present a program for residents and their family members in which they learn to share hand massage with each other. Comfort Touch to the shoulders and/or feet can also be offered.

- **Volunteer coordinator:** A Comfort Touch program might involve a volunteer component. This is particularly true in hospice organizations, because they have a history and mandate of volunteer participation in patient care. A certified massage therapist who is part of the clinical team might instruct selected home care volunteers in the principles of Comfort Touch, along with simple techniques to use with patients.

Private Practice

Many Comfort Touch practitioners work in medical settings as part of their private massage therapy practices. In this case, the therapist is not an employee of a healthcare organization; rather, she or he is reimbursed for services directly by the patient, or the patient's family. The individual is still governed by the local and state requirements for certification, licensing, and insurance. Records of these, along with the individual's resume, references, and tuberculosis test results, should be on file with the facility.

Usually, it is necessary to sign in and out when entering a medical center or other healthcare facility or assisted-living home. It is wise to check in with the nursing staff before a visit to a patient/resident to get an update on your client's condition. Also, after your visit, report to the staff any relevant information that might affect the patient's care. Keep records of your visits, using the CARE Note format.

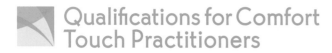

Qualifications for Comfort Touch Practitioners

The practice of Comfort Touch must be consistent with professional standards of healthcare to ensure the safety and well-being of patients in medical settings and residents of nursing facilities. The roles and responsibilities of practitioners might vary somewhat from one organization or facility to another. If the individual has cre-

dentials in another health profession, the practice of Comfort Touch might be incorporated into an existing job. For example, a registered nurse or physical therapist can incorporate awareness of the principles of Comfort Touch, using techniques that are appropriate and complementary to their existing scope of practice.

Comfort Touch practitioners interested in working in medical settings can expect to adhere to the following qualifications, whether to work in medical settings as members of staff, or as independent contract employees. These guidelines will assist both administrators and practitioners in developing successful programs.

- **Training and certification:** Requirements for certification or licensing of massage therapists vary from one locale to another, so check to make sure you are in compliance with state and local regulations. (At the local level, check with the city or county clerk and recorder. At the state level, check with the appropriate state regulatory agencies.) Also, complete the necessary training in Comfort Touch technique before beginning to practice it. Orientation to the specific facility in which services will be provided also should be in compliance with the rules of the organization.
- **Scope of practice:** Observe the scope of practice of your profession, practicing only those skills for which you are trained and/or licensed to practice.
- **Hygiene and Universal Precautions:** Understand and observe all rules of hygiene, including Standard and Universal Precautions. (See Appendix A.)
- **Tuberculosis testing and infectious diseases:** Adhere to the facility's rules regarding tuberculosis testing, and other required immunizations. Do not work if infected with a contagious condition, such as a cold or flu.
- **Professionalism:** Wear clean and appropriate attire, and act in a respectful manner at all times.
- **Timeliness:** Be on time for all appointments or scheduled times of work. Be prompt in returning phone calls regarding setting schedules.
- **Communication and documentation:** Maintain communication with other members of the healthcare team, reporting observations to appropriate supervisors when required. Complete all necessary documentation. (See Chapter 7.)
- **Confidentiality:** To protect the privacy of your clients, observe strict rules of confidentiality. Conversations about clients and written records concerning patients are to be shared only with authorized people who are directly involved in the patients' care.
- **Insurance:** You may be required to carry personal professional liability insurance. Provide

documentation if necessary. If you will be driving to see patients (as in a hospice or home healthcare agency), you will need to show a current driver's license and proof of motor vehicle insurance.

- **Background checks:** Criminal background checks of job applicants are required in most healthcare facilities, particularly for clinical

staff. The applicant may be required to list previous names, addresses of residences, and places of employment.

In developing a program of Comfort Touch, you can use the guidelines listed previously to create a job description for a massage therapist and/or practitioner of Comfort Touch. Figure 9-5 shows an example of a job

---

JOB TITLE: **Massage Therapist/Comfort Touch Practitioner**

REPORTS TO: **Director of Clinical Services**

QUALIFICATIONS:
- Mature individual, supportive of the Hospice concept and willing to complete the Hospice training (30 hours).
- Has certificate of completion (or comparable documentation) showing a minimum of 500 hours of training in massage therapy from a state-approved massage therapy program.
- Proof of professional liability insurance and/or professional affiliation.
- Has completed training in *Comfort Touch* (minimum of 15 hours), and passed written and practical competency tests.
- Willingness and ability to work with a wide variety of clientele and communicate within an interdisciplinary team.
- Ability to be non-judgmental and flexible.
- Ability to communicate with and support others.
- Ability to be reliable and punctual.

SUMMARY OF RESPONSIBILITIES:
The massage therapist provided hands-on comfort care to patients and/or their caregivers. All touch is provided with the intention of providing comfort, and using the principles and techniques outlined in the Comfort Touch training. The massage therapist may incorporate other skills for which they are trained into their service, with the approval of the massage therapy supervisor.

SUPERVISION:
Overall supervision by Director of Clinical Services (Director of Nursing) and direct supervision by the Massage Therapy Supervisor.

PERFORMANCE RESPONSIBILITIES:
- Provides hands-on comfort care to patients and/or their caregiver, using principles and techniques outlined in the Comfort Touch training.
- Provides massage therapy or other modalities of healing or bodywork, as per their training, and as is appropriate for the patient and/or caregiver, with the approval of massage therapy supervisor.
- Maintains communication with other team members on a case, reporting observations or events to case manager (nurse or social worker) and/or massage therapy supervisor when needed.
- Attends interdisciplinary team meetings as required.
- Maintains confidentiality at all times.
- Participates in educational in-services offered by Hospice (at least 2 per year).
- Submits time records to human resources director on a monthly basis.
- Maintains all required patient documentation and submits to clinical services staff on a weekly basis. Documents massage therapy and Comfort Touch sessions using the CARE Note format.
- Meets all health and regulatory requirements of volunteers as interpreted by Hospice, including annual TB tests.
- Keeps staff informed of availability on a regular basis.

Signature of Applicant _____ Date: _____

FIGURE 9-5. Massage therapist job description.

Hints for Practice

Visioning and Setting Goals

Are you an individual massage therapist or healthcare practitioner who is interested in sharing the skills of Comfort Touch with people in healthcare settings? Are you wondering how and where to begin? While it is important to have adequate training in the modality itself, it is also important to clarify your vision of the work you want to do, and to formulate a plan to implement your vision.

Sit down with paper and pen in hand and write as you consider the following:

- Make a list of your current talents, aptitudes, interests, and skills relating to your practice of Comfort Touch.
- Envision whom you want to see as your clients. Do you have experience with this clientele already?
- Envision the setting(s) in which you want to work. Have you visited this setting? What do you know about it?
- Envision the people you wish to see as your co-workers and peers. Do you have any contacts with people you would like to work with as coworkers and/or peers?
- Do you want to work as an independent contractor or a paid employee? Do you want to offer volunteer service in order to gain experience?
- Make a list of the steps you intend to take toward implementing your vision. For example, list any training you intend to take; the people you want to interview; the facilities you wish to visit; the marketing brochure you will make. Set a timeframe to implement each of these actions.

Visioning and goal setting are the initial steps of any new endeavor. The more focused your vision, the easier it will be to implement. If something isn't yielding results, don't hesitate to make adjustments to your plan when and where necessary. Also, understand that as you take deliberate action, new opportunities will present themselves. Go where the energy is!

---

description used in a hospice setting. This form can be adapted to meet the needs of your own organization.

 ## Program Proposals and Funding Options

The development of a Comfort Touch proposal begins with a written document that outlines the intention of the program, and includes guidelines for its implementation within the healthcare organization. It should be presented to the individual(s) in charge of programs and funding for the organization (e.g., an executive director and/or a director of clinical services). It may need approval of an executive board of directors, in accordance with the structure of the organization. A proposal to implement the practice of Comfort Touch needs to include a rationale for providing the service, a suggested organizational/administrative structure for the program, and suggested options for funding.

Rationale for Providing This Service

Describe the benefits of Comfort Touch and how it will enhance the quality of clinical care for the specific population being served in the facility. Describe the charac-teristics that make Comfort Touch a safe, appropriate, and effective complementary therapy in the medical setting or facility. (See Chapter 1.)

Organizational Structure of the Program

Describe how the program will be administered and supervised. Describe the qualifications and roles of practitioners, and specify who will provide initial training and ongoing supervision. Specify who will be in charge of scheduling, documentation, and billing.

Funding

Funding a Comfort Touch program can present a challenge, as there is typically little or no insurance reimbursement for massage therapy in most healthcare settings. However, as more scientific research continue to demonstrate the efficacy of touch therapies, the likelihood of funding options will increase. Meanwhile, existing programs are being funded in a variety of ways. A combination of different approaches can also be implemented to meet the needs and circumstances of a particular organization. For example, some programs offer initial sessions (1–3) to patients free of charge, followed by optional sessions per set fee.

Fee for Service

Touch therapies can be paid for directly by the patient or patient's family, in accordance with agreed-upon fees. Fees are generally in keeping with the hourly rates per massage sessions in the community. A sliding-scale fee, involving discounts based on need, can be used to accommodate a patient's ability to pay. In some settings it may be appropriate for touch sessions to be paid for through the purchase of gift certificates.

Contracts for Hourly Rates

In this option the facility contracts with the Comfort Touch practitioner—either as an independent contractor or as a part-time employee—for a set number of hours on a regular schedule (eg, 4 hours per day, 3 days a week). The facility schedules clients during those times. With this option, payment for the time is guaranteed to the therapist, no matter the number of clients scheduled. If there are more clients scheduled on a particular date, the sessions can be shorter to accommodate more people. This option allows for open scheduling, in which the timing of sessions can be flexible based on demand during a given day.

With this option payment is provided from general patient/client services funds, or from specific monies earmarked for complementary therapies.

Grants/Scholarships

Money to finance a Comfort Touch program can derive from funds raised through specific or general fund-raising activities of the organization. Or it may be derived through charitable grants from individuals or community businesses or organizations.

Research

In some cases, Comfort Touch is provided to patients as part of research studies. Research studies for massage therapy in medical settings may be funded by different entities, including those operating through the National Institutes of Health. Some research is funded by massage-related organizations, educational institutions, and businesses. This is one way to initiate a program that would later need to be sustained through other funding sources.

Student Fieldwork Practicums

Also called internships or externships, student fieldwork practicums are unpaid educational opportunities for qualified students of massage therapy to practice Comfort Touch in a medical setting. They require a high degree of commitment from the educational institution (the massage school), and cooperation with the healthcare organization. Students must meet all the requirements for practice established by the facility, and must be supervised by a qualified massage therapist or other healthcare professional with training in Comfort Touch in the medical setting. Some facilities only allow students to work with staff and/or family members, while others extend the opportunity to work directly with patients.

The structure of an internship can also be approached as a continuing education opportunity for certified massage therapists who are interested in acquiring experience through practicing massage in a medical setting.

Employee Wellness Programs

Comfort Touch can be offered and funded through existing employee wellness programs. Often in the form of 20- to 30-minute sessions of touch in the seated position, this opportunity can be a way for Comfort Touch practitioners to offer the benefits of touch to the staff. It is a good starting place to educate staff members about the benefits of Comfort Touch for patients. Staff can be seated in their own office chairs as they receive the sequence of touch in the seated position (outlined in Chapter 5) with additional emphasis on tonic acupressure points.

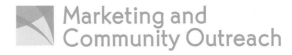

Marketing and Community Outreach

Whether you are an administrator of a touch therapies program or an individual massage therapist, it is important to let others know of your program and the skills you wish to offer. The following are suggestions for educating others within your own organization or to the public at large about these services.

Presentations to Clinical and Administrative Staff

Give a talk for clinical and administrative staff outlining the benefits of Comfort Touch for patients and the residents of the facility. If you have an existing program, explain how it works. If you are proposing a program, paint a picture of how the program can work, citing examples of other successful programs.

In-Services for the Clinical Staff

An in-service to clinical staff can include an introduction to the principles of Comfort Touch, with a simple

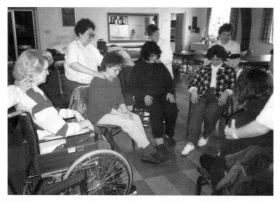

FIGURE 9-6. Comfort Touch In-service. Members of a nursing staff practice Comfort Touch during an in-service training. In-services provide an effective and enjoyable way to introduce staff members to the principles and techniques of Comfort Touch as they share the direct benefits of the work with each other.

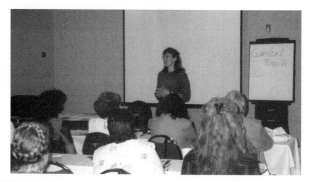

FIGURE 9-7. Community Outreach. Speaking to health organizations and community groups provides an avenue to educate the public about the benefits of Comfort Touch. Public talks can incorporate the use of hands-on demonstrations, and simple hands-on exercises to be shared among the attendees.

demonstration of basic skills. Participants will enjoy a hands-on learning experience that includes a simple exchange of shoulder or hand massage, using basic techniques of Comfort Touch (Figure 9-6).

Articles for Staff and Community

Comfort Touch practitioners can submit short stories of their experiences and successes in their practices to in-house newsletters and journals. Sometimes local newspapers in the community are interested in including news of complementary therapies in a medical setting.

It is also useful to keep a file of published articles regarding research about the benefits of touch. Use these and other written or video resources when giving presentations.

Public Speaking and Community Outreach

Local service organizations and community health organizations are often interested in learning about new and innovative programs offered in healthcare facilities. Many special interest groups host guest speakers to share information of interest to their members. Consider speaking about the benefits of Comfort Touch to staff and clientele of senior centers and retirement homes; family caregivers of the elderly; members of support groups for people with such conditions as diabetes, cancer, Alzheimer disease, Parkinson disease, etc. It is always best to include a simple demonstration. As with in-services, audiences can enjoy a simple exchange of hands-on skills (Figure 9-7).

Networking

Never underestimate the value of connecting with other people and talking about your work, whether they are healthcare professionals or interested individuals. Opportunities for change and innovation happen because of individuals, not because of institutions. Nurture relationships with people who are interested in the inherent value of this work. It is not necessary to "hard sell" Comfort Touch, because this work relates to basic universal human needs and desires. Do not spend too much time trying to convince people who do not indicate interest. Sometimes it is only necessary to plant a seed, and let it grow in its own time.

STORY

Meet Me Here

"I've got rocks in my head," Agnes would say to her caregivers at the nursing home. Her words were usually attributed to a confused state of mind that resulted from Alzheimer disease. No one understood the 94-year-old woman when she complained, "The rockets are taking off in my head!"

Ron Baggett, a massage therapist employed by a hospice in Kansas City, Missouri, was assigned to see Agnes. "She was very wary as I started the first session, but within a few seconds of touching her shoulders her expression warmed and our friendship began."

Ron discovered that her reference to "rocks in her head" was her way of conveying that her head felt too heavy to hold up. "The rockets taking off" described the neck spasms that jerked her neck with an audible click, sending popping sensations along her spine.

Agnes rarely recognized members of her own family or the nursing staff who cared for her daily, but after that initial session with Ron, she always recognized him and knew his name. She commented to others about

"Ron, the back doctor," and how he helped her to manage the "rocks" in her head. Ron continued to see her, offering comforting touch, for nearly 9 months. Her response was always appreciative.

He was surprised one day, however, when she didn't recognize him as he walked into her room. But when he touched her, he noted the familiar spark in her eye, as she broke into a smile, saying, "Oh, it's you."

She sighed gratefully as he proceeded to work with her. As he ended the session, Agnes grabbed his hand, looked him straight in the eye, speaking earnestly, "I want you to meet me here next week."

"Of course, I'll see you next week," he assured her.

"No," she shook her head and placed her left hand over her heart. Agnes was tapping her chest as she spoke, "I want you to meet me <u>here</u> next week. Do you hear me?"

Ron smiled and said, "Yes, I do hear you." He gently squeezed her hand, then touched her head softly with one hand. He pointed to his own heart and added, "I'll meet you right here."

During that week Ron waited to hear of Agnes' condition. On the day of their next scheduled visit, he learned that she had died peacefully in her sleep early that morning. Later, as Ron reflected on his experience with her, he said, "Agnes taught me a lot about letting my work become what the patient needs it to be."

Ron's willingness to truly listen to his client, coupled with a clear intention to offer comfort through touch, made this interaction a powerful healing experience for both of them.

Summary

- As a complementary therapy, Comfort Touch can safely and easily be incorporated into any healthcare setting as an adjunct to conventional medicine and nursing care.
- Comfort Touch programs can be administered in a variety of ways, depending on the focus of care for the client population, the setting of the facility, and the management structure of the healthcare organization.
- The qualifications of Comfort Touch practitioners should be consistent with the professional standards of healthcare, to ensure the safety and well-being of patients in medical settings and homecare, and the residents of nursing and assisted-living facilities. These qualifications include proper training and certification, understanding of the rules of hygiene, adherence to required medical tests and/or immunizations, communication with the healthcare team,

and completion of the required patient care documentation (CARE Notes).
- The development of a Comfort Touch program can begin with a written proposal outlining the following: the rationale for providing the service; a proposed administrative structure for the program; and options for funding.
- Funding for a Comfort Touch program can include a variety of options, ranging from fee for service to a practitioner who is an independent contractor, to funding based on status as a part-time or full-time employee of a healthcare organization.
- As an administrator of a program or a practitioner of Comfort Touch, it is important to inform others within your organization of the scope of the program and its benefits for patients. Likewise, community outreach helps educate the public about the benefits of touch as a valuable complementary therapy for the elderly and for those in medical settings.

Review Questions

1. List the names of four to six medical centers and/or residential facilities for the elderly in your area.
2. Describe how you would convey the benefits of a Comfort Touch program to an administrator of a medical facility.
3. List several qualifications for a practitioner of Comfort Touch.
4. What is meant by "scope of practice?"
5. Describe the administrative structure you would prefer to be involved in as an administrator and as a practitioner of Comfort Touch.
6. In your circumstance, what do you envision as the primary vehicle for funding a program of Comfort Touch?
7. Name three or four organizations or groups in your community that might be interested in learning about the benefits of Comfort Touch. How would you go about learning more about one of them in order to make contact?
8. Describe the value of networking as you promote a program of Comfort Touch.

Suggested Reading

Corbin L. Safety and efficacy of massage therapy for patients with cancer. *Cancer Control.* 2005; July: pp 158–164.

Moyer CA, Rounds J, Hannum JW. A meta-analysis of massage therapy research. *Psychological Bulletin.* 2004; 130(1), 3–18.

Sohnen-Moe CM. *Business Mastery, Fourth Edition: A Guide for Creating a Fulfilling, Thriving Business and Keeping It Successful.* Tucson: Sohnen-Moe Associates; 2007.

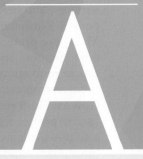

Infection Control: Standard and Universal Precautions

All healthcare providers are required to understand and observe necessary rules of hygiene to prevent the spread of disease. Observance of these rules protects both patients and healthcare workers. **Standard Precautions** are guidelines adopted by the Centers for Disease Control and Prevention that are designed to reduce the risk of transmission of microorganisms from both recognized and unrecognized sources of infection in hospitals and other medical settings. Standard Precautions synthesize the major features of **Universal Precautions** (blood and body fluid precautions) and body substance isolation (pathogens from moist body surfaces).

If you are a massage therapist or Comfort Touch practitioner working in a medical setting, you will be required to learn these precautions. With all due concern for observance of these precautions to avoid the spread of infection, it is still possible to provide a quality experience of touch for the patient. Check with your supervisor if you have questions about when to use personal protection equipment such as gloves, masks, or gowns. Even if you are wearing a mask or gloves, the techniques of Comfort Touch can be offered safely and effectively.

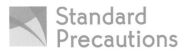

Standard Precautions

These are the basic level of infection control that should be used in the care of all patients all of the time. They are used to reduce the risk of transmission of micro-

organisms from both recognized and non-recognized sources of infection. They apply to:

- Blood
- All body fluids
- Secretions and excretions (except sweat), whether or not they contain visible blood
- Non-intact skin
- Mucous membranes

Personal protective equipment (PPE) to carry out Standard Precautions include:

- Gowns
- Masks
- Eye protection
- Face shield (if splashes or sprays of blood or body fluids is likely)

Standard Precautions include:

- **Hand hygiene:** Wash hands for 20 seconds with soap and warm water, before and after patient contact. (Remember to keep fingernails short and clean.) Wash hands after touching blood, body fluids, excretions, and contaminated items, whether or not gloves are worn.
- **Gloves:** Wear clean, nonsterile gloves when touching or coming into contact with blood, body fluids, secretions, or excretions. Remove gloves promptly after use and discard before touching noncontaminated items or environmental

surfaces, and before providing care to another patient. Wash hands after removing gloves.

- **Mask, eye protection, face shield:** Protect eyes, nose, mouth, and mucous membranes from exposure to sprays or splashes of blood, body fluids, secretions, and excretions.
- **Gowns:** Fluid resistant, non-sterile gowns are used to protect against soiling of clothing during activities that may generate splashes or sprays of blood, body fluids, secretions, or excretions.
- **Patient-care equipment:** Handle soiled patient-care equipment, including linens, in a manner that prevents skin and mucous membrane exposure, contamination of clothing, and transfer of microorganisms to other patients and environments. Clean, disinfect, or reprocess nondisposable equipment before reuse with another patient. Discard single-use items properly. Take care to prevent injuries when handling needles, scalpels, and other sharp instruments or devices. Place disposable syringes and other sharp items in appropriate puncture-resistance containers.

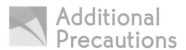

Additional Precautions

There are additional measures that can be taken, when appropriate, to reduce the spread of infection. Standard Precautions always apply as the basic level of infection control.

- **Contact Precautions:** These are used in the care of patients known or suspected to have a serious illness easily transmitted by direct patient contact or by indirect contact with items in the patient's environment. In addition to Standard Precautions, Contact Precautions include the use of a private patient room, with additional care given to the use of gloves and gowns for workers when entering and providing care in the patient's room. Particular care must also be taken with patient transport out of the room, and with patient-care equipment.
- **Droplet Precautions:** Droplets can be generated during coughing, sneezing, talking, and during certain medical procedures, such as suctioning. Droplets may contain microorganisms and generally travel no more than 3 feet from the patient. These droplets can be deposited on the host's nasal mucosa, conjunctiva, or mouth. In addition to Standard Precautions, wear a surgical mask when working within 3 feet of the patient. In addition, it is recommended that the patient be placed in a private room, with care taken upon patient transport.
- **Airborne Precautions:** Airborne pathogens are microorganisms that are much smaller than droplets, and can remain suspended in the air for long periods of time. These microorganisms can be dispersed widely by air currents and may become inhaled or deposited on a susceptible host within the same room or over a longer distance from the source patient, depending on environmental factors. Therefore, special air handling and ventilation are required to prevent airborne transmission. Standard Precautions are used in patient care, with additional respiratory protection for healthcare workers. Patients should be in private rooms, with special care provided on patient transport.

Integrating Aroma:
Cautions and Considerations

The practice of therapeutic touch has long had an association with the use of oils and scents. Traditionally, massage practitioners use oils or lotions on the skin to allay the friction created by certain gliding or kneading techniques and to moisturize the skin. Scents, in the form of essential oils, are often incorporated into these oils for aesthetic and therapeutic benefits. Essential oils are also used in candles, air fresheners, and water-based sprays that diffuse scent into the room.

The practice of Comfort Touch does not require the use of lotions or oils, because it is based on broad, encompassing techniques of acupressure that do not cause friction on the skin. It is also usually practiced on a client who is clothed, so the use of oils on the skin is not practical. But many massage therapists are accustomed to and/or drawn to the use of fragrances in their practice of touch therapies, so the question arises, "Is it beneficial and/or safe to incorporate the use of aroma into the practice of Comfort Touch?"

 ## Causes for Concern

It is important to recognize some of the problems and concerns associated with the use of scents. Many of the substances used in popular scented products are synthetic chemicals with known detrimental effects. There is also cause for concern when using products that are listed as having natural or organic ingredients. Essential

oils derived from plants, whether organically grown or not, are highly concentrated substances, requiring 20 to 100 ounces of plant material to produce an ounce of essential oil. Strongly scented essential oils can mask rancidity in carrier oils, such as almond or sunflower.

Allergies, Sensitivities, and Irritation

The primary cause for concern in the use of scents is the potential for allergies, sensitivities, and irritation. Whether the scents are derived from synthetic chemicals or essential oils distilled from whole plants, many people are sensitive to the effects of these substances, whether they are airborne or applied to the skin. The user of essential oils must always be alert to the possibility of allergic reactions. Sensitivities may develop over time and can be especially hard to identify if a variety of essential oils are used in combination. Allergies can manifest as sneezing, itchy eyes, headaches, dizziness, skin irritation or rashes, or severe respiratory distress.

In working with the elderly and the chronically ill, the touch therapist should be especially sensitive to the fact that many in this population already have compromised respiratory and/or immune function, so allergies and sensitivities to scent can be a critical issue. Some in this population also have limited ability to communicate verbally, so might have more difficulty in communicating their needs regarding scent.

Individual Needs and Preferences

Exposure to a particular scent, with its complex chemical components, can trigger associations to prior experience. It can remind us of a person, place, an event, or a particular substance or emotional response. The person's reaction can be positive and uplifting if the association is a pleasant one, but it can also be evocative of disagreeable feelings if the association is not favorable. For this reason, it is best not to assume that a particular scent will affect one person in the same manner it affects another. Also, remember that it is our primary intention to comfort the people we touch. Avoid projecting your own preferences on your clients, or trying to treat them using the purported benefits of a particular scented product.

Desensitization of the Sense of Smell

Frequent use of essential oils can result in desensitization, the loss of responsiveness to smell. For example, a massage therapist who uses a particular essential oil regularly, whether on her or his own body or in the practice of massage, may gradually lose the ability to smell the full intensity of that aroma. This can lead to even greater use of the scent, with the unintended consequence of imposing that scent on others.

The human sense of smell is designed to discern many different scents. One should be able to tell if a food is fresh or rancid, desirable, or undesirable. One should be able to distinguish one substance from another. The well-developed sense of smell can help us to identify particular plants in the wild or in the garden. Smell is one of the methods by which a mother and a baby bond. Scent can attract people to each other, and it can repel people from each other. The sense of smell alerts us to danger, as in the smell of a gas leak or a fire, or other toxic substances in the environment.

Overuse of essential oils, or other strongly scented substances, diminishes our ability to use our sense of smell to its full potential. Ultimately, this can also diminish our enjoyment of the full range of pleasurable scents available to us.

Cleanliness

Remember the importance of good personal hygiene, and avoid the use of strong scents on your own body. Strive to create and maintain a clean environment in which you work. It is preferable to use unscented cleaning products. You might want to open windows or doors between sessions to bring fresh air into the room.

 # Using Scents Sensibly

Given the cautions mentioned previously, we can consider ways in which it might be appropriate to incorporate the use of aroma into the practice of massage. There is no doubt that exposure to aroma can enhance our enjoyment of life. The smell of fresh flowers and fragrant greens are uplifting and pleasant to many people. The herbs and spices used in cooking are the everyday **natural scent therapy** of many traditions, adding flavor to food, awakening the senses, and stimulating digestive juices. A cup of steaming herbal tea can prompt one to take a deep breath, inhaling the volatile oils of the herb.

Here are some suggestions for ways to safely integrate aroma into a massage therapy practice:

- **Use live plants or fresh flowers:** Notice the scents of live plants if you have a garden. Bring a few stems of fresh lavender or a small bouquet of roses or carnations to your massage sessions. Not only will the scent be likely to delight your clients, but the color and sight of the plants or flower will enhance the quality of the atmosphere you are creating.
- **Use dried flowers:** For example, a sprig of lavender stems and flowers tied with a ribbon is a delightful addition to the décor of a room, subtly imparting its scent over time. A basket of rose petals is a beautiful sight, as well as a sensual aromatic treat to many people.
- **Use coconut oil:** Natural coconut oil is a stable oil that is more resistant to rancidity than most other common oils. It melts at 76°C, has a very light smooth texture, and has a scent that is often considered pleasant. It can be used as a nurturing oil on dry skin.
- **Use infused oil for skin care:** Whole plant material can be infused in pure olive oil (which is a very stable oil), to extract its medicinal qualities, and to impart its scent. Use aromatic fresh plant material that has been allowed to dry for a few days. For example, place finely chopped lavender leaves in a jar; fill it with pure olive oil, and cap it with a canning lid so that no air gets in. Let it sit on the counter out of sunlight for 2 to 3 weeks. Do not refrigerate. Room temperature is necessary to the process. Strain the oil through a handkerchief and store in a cool, dry place. It can be left unrefrigerated for several weeks, or it will keep for several months to a year in the refrigerator. Other plants that can be used include: big sagebrush (*artemisia tridentata*), rosemary, lemon balsam, or fresh St. John's wort flowers (*hypericum perforatum*).

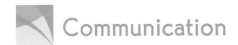
Communication

If you incorporate the use of scent in your practice, be sure to check with your clients to make sure that any oil or other scented material you use is acceptable to them. Even fresh flowers can be too much for some people, particularly if they have respiratory conditions such as asthma, COPD, or hayfever-type allergies. Honor the client's needs and preferences. If the client requests that you use a special scented lotion of his or her own, you can honor that request, if it is acceptable to you.

Recommended Resources: An Annotated List

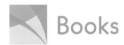 Books

Beers MH, Berkow R, eds. *The Merck Manual of Geriatrics.* 3rd ed. Whitehouse Station, NJ: Merck & Company; 2000. The Merck Manual of Geriatrics is a comprehensive, thumb-indexed handbook detailing an interdisciplinary approach to care of the elderly. Currently out of print, but still in distribution, the content is available and continuously updated online at www.merck.com.

Bowden B, Bowden J. *An Illustrated Atlas of the Skeletal Muscles.* 2nd ed. Englewood, CO: Morton Publishing Company; 2005. A useful reference guide indicating the location of the motor points (referred to in the text as "trigger points") of the skeletal muscles.

Brooke E. *Medicine Women: A Pictorial History of Women Healers.* Wheaton, IL: Quest Books; 1997. In this fascinating history of women healers, Elizabeth Brooke explores their role in various historical and cultural contexts. This book provides a context to understand the traditions of healing from the primary caregiving role of women, through the development of high-tech medicine to the resurgence of interest in holistic medical treatment, with its emphasis on providing care through nurturing touch.

Callahan M, Kelley P. *Final Gifts: Understanding the Special Awareness, Needs and Communications of the Dying.* New York, NY: Bantam Books; 1992. Hospice nurses Maggie Callahan and Patricia Kelley share the richness of their experience in tending to the terminally ill. They recount stories of the ways in which the dying patients communicate their needs, reveal their feelings, and even choreograph their final moments. This inspiring book offers helpful advice to all caregivers on the art of listening with compassion, enhancing the quality of experience for all concerned.

Curties D. *Breast Massage.* Moncton, NB: Curties-Overzet Publications; 1999. Massage educator Debra Curties explains the anatomy and physiology of the female breast, and establishes safe protocols for the practice of therapeutic breast massage. She describes techniques that are used to treat post-surgical scarring, ease the discomforts of pregnancy and breastfeeding, and to alleviate the congestion and edema which cause breast pain. She teaches that massage therapists can play a role in supporting their clients' regular breast monitoring practices.

Davis MS. *Caring in Remembered Ways.* Blue Hill, ME: Heartsong Books; 1999. This inspiring memoir by Maggie Steincrohn Davis is filled with stories emphasizing the importance of caregiving as an essential part of meaningful human interaction.

Duff K. *The Alchemy of Illness.* New York, NY: Bell Tower; 1993. Drawing from her experience with chronic fatigue syndrome, counselor Kat Duff offers acknowledgement and inspiration to people suffering from chronic illnesses. It offers useful insights and lessons in compassion for caregivers.

Dunn H. *Hard Choices For Loving People: CPR, Artificial Feeding, Comfort Care and the Patient with a Life-Threatening Illness.* 4th ed. Herndon, VA: A & A Publishers; 2001. This booklet by chaplain Hank Dunn is written for people who are making medical treatment decisions in the face of life-threatening illness. He discusses the issues involved when considering the use or cessation of life-prolonging treatments (such as cardiopulmonary resuscitation (CPR), artificial hydration and nutrition, antibiotics use, etc.) versus the use of "comfort measures only."

Dunn T, Williams M. *Massage Therapy Guidelines for Hospital and Home Care,* 4th ed. Olympia, WA: Information for People; 2000. This manual was written and compiled by Tedi Dunn and Marian Williams, pioneers in the development of hospital-based massage programs. It is a resource for bodyworkers, administrators, and massage educators. They draw on the wisdom and experience of other notable people in the field, including Karen Gibson, Irene Smith, Dawn Nelson, Gayle MacDonald, and Laura Koch.

Feil N. *The Validation Breakthrough: Simple Techniques for Communicating with People With "Alzheimer's-Type Dementia."* 2nd ed. Baltimore, MD: Health Professions Press; 2002. The simple and practical communication techniques developed by internationally recognized expert Naomi Feil have helped thousands of professional and family caregivers to improve their relationships with confused clients or loved ones and to understand and handle challenging behaviors.

Foster MA. *Somatic Patterning: How to Improve Posture and Movement and Ease Pain.* Longmont, CO: EMS Press; 2007. In this richly illustrated sourcebook, Mary Ann Foster shares her extensive knowledge of somatic patterning, a therapeutic modality that works to change harmful or inefficient body-use patterns using awareness and movement as primary tools.

Frank A. *At the Will of the Body – Reflections on Illness.* Boston, MA: Houghton Mifflin; 1991. Arthur Frank draws on his own experience with life-threatening illnesses—heart disease and cancer—to explore the meaning of life, while offering many insights for caregivers.

Gach MR. *Acupressure's Potent Points: A Guide to Self-Care for Common Ailments.* New York, NY: Bantam Books; 1990. This reference guide to acupressure points by Michael Reed Gach includes over 500 illustrations and photos showing how to find potent points used in traditional acupressure to help relieve a myriad of ailments from headaches and muscular pain to nausea and fatigue.

Greene E, Goodrich-Dunn B. *The Psychology of the Body.* Baltimore, MD: Lippincott Williams & Wilkins; 2004. Elliot Greene and Barbara Goodrich-Dunn explore the intricate connections between the mind and the body and the underlying psychological factors that influence the massage therapist–client relationship. This text gives practical guidance to assist bodyworkers in understanding and responding appropriately to the emotional issues of their clients.

Hass E. *Staying Healthy With the Seasons.* Berkeley, CA: Celestial Arts; 2003. This classic of integrative medicine, written by physician Elson Haas and originally published in 1981, is a balanced blend of Eastern and Western medicines, nutrition, herbology, exercise, and a wealth of other health topics. It has a clear and concise introduction to the applications of traditional Chinese medical theory.

Holmes J. *John Bowlby and Attachment Theory.* London, UK: Routledge; 1993. Jeremy Holmes explores the work of John Bowlby whose formulation of Attachment Theory—the propensity of humans to form affectional bonds and the consequences of their loss and disruption—has greatly influenced the field of developmental psychology.

Juhan D. *Job's Body: A Handbook for Bodywork.* 3rd ed. Barrytown, NY: Station Hill Press; 2003. Deane Juhan examines the physiology and psychology of the human response to touch, combining excellent illustrations with a detailed but readable technical discussion.

Kubler-Ross E. *On Death and Dying.* New York, NY: Touchstone; 1969. This classic work by noted physician and psychiatrist Elizabeth Kubler-Ross, explores the now-famous psychological stages of death: denial, anger, bargaining, depression and acceptance. Her work greatly influenced the development of the hospice movement, and laid a foundation for the subsequent study of the psychosocial aspects of coping with chronic illness and dying.

MacDonald G. *Massage for the Hospital Patient and Medically Frail Client.* Baltimore, MD: Lippincott Williams & Wilkins; 2005. Gayle MacDonald provides a valuable resource text for massage therapists, health professionals, and administrators wanting practical information to assist in developing programs of safe, effective massage therapy as part of complementary care in medical settings.

MacDonald G. *Medicine Hands: Massage Therapy for People with Cancer.* 2nd ed. Forres, Scotland: Findhorn Press; 2007. Gayle MacDonald deconstructs common myths about the use of massage in cancer treatment, and stresses that the real issues for massage therapists center on supporting the cancer patient with the benefits of appropriate massage while ameliorating the discomforts of medical treatments.

McIntosh N. *The Educated Heart: Professional Boundaries for Massage Therapists, Bodyworkers, and Movement Teachers.* 2nd ed. Baltimore, MD: Lippincott Williams & Wilkins; 2005. This handbook offers guidance for understanding relationship dynamics and establishing professional and ethical boundaries in client–therapist interactions. Replete with real-life examples, Nina McIntosh presents practical solutions to sensitive situations including confidentiality, sexual attraction, socializing with clients, and negotiating fees.

Montague A. *Touching: The Human Significance of Skin.* 3rd ed. New York, NY: Harper & Row; 1986. A groundbreaking work first published in 1971, this book provides a compelling examination of the importance of tactile interaction—touching—on all facets of human development. Anthropologist Dr. Ashley Montague draws attention to the skin and the effect of touching on mental and physical health. He devotes a chapter to the importance of touching for older people.

Nelson D. *From the Heart Through the Hands: The Power of Touch in Caregiving.* Forres, Scotland: Findhorn Press; 2006. Both inspirational and informative, this text by massage therapist Dawn Nelson is a compilation of her knowledge gleaned from many years of experience as a hands-on caregiver.

Nelson D. *Making Friends With Cancer.* Forres, Scotland: Findhorn Press; 2000. This is Dawn Nelson's personal story, facing the fears and challenges of living with and surviving a diagnosis of cancer. She urges the reader to make informed choices and conscious commitments to live in the present moment.

Pert C. *Molecules of Emotion: The Science Behind Body–Mind Medicine.* New York, NY: Simon and Schuster; 1997. Candace Pert, a research scientist, recounts her work in developing an understanding of the biomolecular basis for emotions. Her work furthers the scientific basis for understanding the link between the body and the mind.

Rando T. *How To Go On Living When Someone You Love Dies.* New York, NY: Bantam; 1991. Clinical psychologist Therese A. Rando brings understanding to the experience of grieving, outlining common phases in the process. She emphasizes that different people respond to loss in different ways, and provides practical tools to assist others to move from acknowledging and experiencing the pain of loss to adapting into a new life reality.

Rose MK. *Bereavement: Dealing with Grief and Loss.* Longmont, CO: Wild Rose; 1996. This booklet is a concise guide to understanding the grieving process. It discusses the losses for which a person mourns, describes different aspects of the cycle of grief, and gives helpful suggestions for coping with the stress of loss. It suggests practical ways for friends and caregivers to support bereaved individuals who are dealing with loss.

Smith I. *Providing Massage in Hospice Care: An Everflowing Resource.* San Francisco, CA: Everflowing; 2007. *Everflowing* is a modality of bodywork developed by Irene Smith, a leader in the field of massage for the elderly and the chronically ill. This manual represents over twenty years of her experience in developing protocols, skills, and coping strategies for facilitating bodywork with dying persons. It addresses the multidimensional challenges and personal healing nature of this profoundly intimate work.

Thompson G. *Shiatsu: A Complete Step-by-Step Guide.* New York, NY: Sterling Publishing Company; 2000. Illustrated throughout with the beautiful color photography of Sue Atkinson, this practical workbook by Gerry Thompson makes the benefits of the traditional Japanese healing art of Shiatsu accessible to everyone. He emphasizes self-care for the practitioner through correct body alignment, along with simple routines for self-Shiatsu treatment.

Weed S. *Healing Wise—Wise Woman Herbal.* Woodstock, NY: Ash Tree Publishing; 1989. Herbalist and health educator Susun S. Weed explores the major traditions of healing—the scientific (conventional), the heroic (alternative), and the wise woman (nurturing)—defining a context to understand approaches to healthcare and lifestyle. She also enumerates 7 Steps of Healing to guide the individual in making practical healthcare decisions.

Werner R. *Massage Therapist's Guide to Pathology.* 4th ed. Baltimore, MD: Lippincott Williams & Wilkins; 2008. This well-organized and comprehensive text written by Ruth Werner is designed to assist the massage therapist in understanding the pathology of a full range of human diseases and dysfunctions, including the implications of the use of conventional massage for each condition.

Worden JW. *Grief Counseling and Grief Therapy: A Handbook for the Mental Health Practitioner.* 3rd ed. New York, NY: Springer Publishing Company, Inc.; 2004. J. William Worden describes the mechanisms of grief and the procedures for helping clients accomplish the "tasks of mourning" to facilitate moving through the process of normal grieving. While it is written for mental health professionals, it is also useful for allied health professionals and hospice personnel who facilitate bereavement support groups.

 ## Video/DVD

Hedley G. *The Integral Anatomy Series: Vol. 1: Skin and Superficial Fascia* [DVD]. New Paltz, NY: Integral Anatomy Productions; 2005. In this video production anatomist Gil Hedley offers the viewer rare visions into the inner layers of the human skin and superficial fascia. These stunning images inspire the hands-on therapist with valuable new insights and information about the living bodies they touch.

Rose M. *Comfort Touch—Massage for the Elderly and the Ill* [Video/DVD and 40-page written guide]. Boulder, CO: Wild Rose; 2004. This video provides a practical introduction to the principles and techniques of *Comfort Touch*®, a nurturing form of acupressure that is safe and appropriate for the elderly and the ill. The author shares the essential elements of this work with demonstrations of its application with clients in the seated, supine, and side-lying positions.

 ## Websites

http://nccam.nih.gov. The National Center for Complementary and Alternative Medicine (NCCAM) is the Federal Government's lead agency for scientific research on complementary and alternative medicine (CAM). They disseminate authoritative information to the public and professionals.

www.comforttouch.com. This is the educational site for information about Comfort Touch®, nurturing acupressure for the elderly and the ill. It includes information about the principles and techniques of Comfort Touch®, trainings, resources, and featured articles.

www.hbmn.com. Founded by Laura Koch, the Hospital-Based Massage Network supports massage and touch therapists pursuing integration of complementary care into mainstream medicine through their work.

www.nhpco.org. The National Hospice and Palliative Care Organization (NHPCO) is the largest nonprofit membership organization representing hospice and palliative care programs and professionals in the United States. Through educational programs and materials, the organization is committed to improving end-of-life care and expanding access to hospice and palliative care.

A

Acupressure An approach to bodywork based on an understanding of the meridians or pathways of energy identified in traditional Chinese medicine and acupuncture. Pressure is applied along the meridians and to specific points, called "tsubo," found along these pathways.

Acute illness Sudden and/or short-term illness or presentation of symptoms; if symptoms persist, may develop into chronic illness or disability.

Aging A process of gradual and spontaneous change, resulting in maturation through childhood, puberty, and young adulthood and then decline through middle and late age.

AIDS Acquired immune deficiency syndrome is a disease of cellular immunodeficiency resulting from infection with the human immunodeficiency virus (HIV). It is characterized by opportunistic infections. It is transmitted from person to person via bodily fluids (blood, semen, vaginal fluid, and breast milk).

Alternative medicine Therapeutic practices that are used *in place of* conventional medicine. An example of an alternative therapy is the use of a special diet to treat cancer instead of undergoing surgery, radiation, or chemotherapy that might be recommended by a conventional doctor.

Alzheimer disease A degenerative disorder of the brain, it involves shrinkage and death of neural tissue. Most common in people over the age of 65, it causes memory loss, personality changes, disorientation, and eventual loss of physical function leading to death.

Amyotrophic lateral sclerosis Also known as Lou Gehrig's disease or ALS, it is a progressive condition that destroys motor neurons in the central and peripheral nervous system, leading to the atrophy of voluntary muscles. Loss of autonomic muscle function often leads to loss of respiratory function.

Atherosclerosis A hardening of the arteries resulting from the accumulation of fatty deposits along the arterial walls.

B

Bereavement is the process of mourning—the response to loss—in which an individual might experience a range of physical, mental, and emotional reactions, including but not limited to sadness, fear, regret, and yearning for whom or what was lost.

Body energy therapies Also called *energy medicine* or *vibrational healing*, these modalities are based on an understanding and awareness of subtle energy that surrounds and permeates the human body. This energy is referred to by various names, including chi, ki, prana, etheric energy, aura field, chakras, and orgone. Body energy therapies derive from many cultural and spiritual healing traditions and include Qigong, Johrei, Reiki, Therapeutic Touch, Polarity Therapy, Healing Touch, Attunement, and prayer. Techniques involve light touch or hands held a few inches from the body of the client, to influence and balance the energy field. Some modalities focus on areas of the body relating to endocrine glands and major organs and nerve plexuses.

Bursitis Inflammation of a bursa, which is a pad-like sac or cavity found in the connective tissue in the area of a joint. Bursas are lined with synovial fluid that acts to reduce friction in areas of movement.

C

CARE Notes Method for documenting massage therapy. Based on a model of narrative charting, it records the **C**ondition of the client, the **A**ction taken, the **R**esponse of the client, and **E**valuation of the session.

Cataracts A leading cause of blindness due to opacity of the lens or capsule of the eye. It can be effectively treated by surgical removal of the affected lens and implantation of a plastic lens.

Cerebral palsy A disease stemming from causes occurring before or during birth, or in early childhood. Those affected have impaired muscle function, with sometimes random involuntary movements.

Cerebrovascular accident (CVA) Sudden loss of consciousness followed by paralysis caused by interference to the blood supply in the brain, resulting from hemorrhage or formation of emboli (blood clots). A CVA can be fatal, or result in significant loss of physical and mental function. Also called **Stroke.**

Chi Chinese word meaning "vital energy," used to describe the flow of energy or life force throughout the body. Also called **ki** in Japanese.

Chronic illness Illness or presentation of symptoms of long-term duration. May begin as an acute illness.

Chronic obstructive pulmonary disease (COPD) A group of diseases, including chronic bronchitis and emphysema, characterized by chronic airflow obstruction.

Client information form A form used to record pertinent information about a person receiving massage therapy. It includes the client's name, contact information, medical history, current health condition, and other information relevant to receiving touch therapy.

Client-centered This is a concept whereby the needs of the client are acknowledged and, whenever possible, influence treatment and communication choices made by the therapist. For example, the client chooses her or his own positioning for the massage session, and the therapist adapts to that. Likewise, conversation is focused primarily on the needs and interests of the client.

Coma Derived from the Greek word *koma,* meaning "deep sleep," it is the profound state of unconsciousness characterized by the absence of eye opening, verbal response, and motor response.

Comfort Touch® A nurturing style of bodywork designed to be safe, appropriate, and effective for use with the elderly and the ill. It follows specific principles that guide the intention of the therapist to comfort the client. Comfort Touch techniques generally rely on broad, full-hand contact which encompasses the part of the body being touched. Pressure is directed perpendicularly into the part of the body being touched, with specific attention given to the appropriate amount of pressure to ensure a sensation that is calming and soothing.

Complementary medicine Therapeutic practices that are designed to nurture the individual physically, mentally, and emotionally. They may be used alone or in conjunction with, and are therefore complementary to, conventional medicine. Examples include massage therapy, nutritional therapy, and music and art therapy. In combination with conventional medicine, these practices may also be referred to as *integrative medicine* or *holistic healing.*

Congestive heart failure Heart condition characterized by diminished blood flow to the tissues of the body, and consequent accumulation of excess blood in the various organs because the heart is unable to pump out the blood returned to it by the great veins. It is usually caused by coronary artery disease.

Connective tissue Provides supporting framework and connection among the parts of the body. Formed of fibrous substance, the bulk of connective tissue is intercellular substance or matrix and, except for cartilage, is highly vascular. Forms of connective tissue include mucous, loose, adipose, fibrous (fascia), lymphoid tissues. Dense connective tissue includes cartilage and bone. Blood and lymph are considered connective tissue, the ground substance of which is a liquid. Epithelium, muscle, and nerve tissue are not connective tissue.

Contracture Static muscle shortening due to tonic spasm or fibrosis; to loss of muscular balance, the antagonists being paralyzed; or to a loss of motion of the adjacent joint.

Conventional massage Dominant form of massage practiced in the Western world, it is based on the strokes of Swedish Massage—effleurage (gliding), petrissage (kneading), friction, vibration, tapotement (percussion), and joint movements. Usually practiced on a client who is lying on a massage table and disrobed but fully draped. The therapist usually uses lotion or oil when performing the massage. See also **Swedish Massage.**

Conventional medicine Dominant form of medicine in the developed world, it involves the use of diagnostic methods and technologies, standards of research or evidence-based practices, and employs the use of pharmaceutical drugs and surgical procedures.

Coronary artery disease Narrowing of the coronary arteries that supply blood to the heart muscle itself. The narrowing is usually caused by atherosclerosis, a hardening of the arteries resulting from accumulation of fatty deposits along the arterial walls.

Cortisol A steroid hormone secreted by the adrenal cortex that is involved in the response to stress; it increases blood pressure and blood sugar levels and suppresses the immune system. It acts as an anti-inflammatory.

Curing Connotes the restoration of someone to a state of health, free from disease or ailment. Curative measures may include appropriate medical interventions, such as surgery or pharmaceutical treatment. Curing, in this sense, requires a diagnosis and an intervention that changes the stated diagnosis. For example, the use of surgery, radiation, and/or chemotherapy, which cures the individual of a malignant tumor.

D

Deep vein thrombosis A blood clot that develops in a deep vein, usually in the leg. This can happen if the vein is damaged or if the flow of blood slows down or stops. It can cause pain in the leg and lead to life-threatening complications if it breaks off and travels via the bloodstream to the lungs.

Diabetes A disease of impaired glucose metabolism that results from inadequate production (Type 1 diabetes—insulin dependent diabetes mellitus) or utilization (Type 2 diabetes—non-insulin dependent diabetes mellitus) of the hormone insulin, a vital substance necessary to convert carbohydrates into energy. Elevated levels of glucose in the blood (hyperglycemia) lead to acute symptoms and long-term complications.

Doula A person trained to give nonmedical support to women who are preparing for birth and to assist during and after the event.

E

Edema An accumulation of an excessive amount of watery fluid in cells or intercellular tissues; swelling.

Empty calories Refers to food that contains caloric content but without appreciable nutrient content.

Endorphin Opioid peptides originally isolated in the brain but also found in many parts of the body. In the nervous system, endorphins bind to the same receptors that bind exogenous opiates, producing pharmacological effects of pain relief and euphoria.

Epinephrine Along with norepinephrine, is a hormone produced by the adrenal glands in response to stress, and is associated with the physiologic responses to fear and anxiety.

Epithelial tissue Cells that line the outer surfaces of the body and line the body cavities. It forms the secreting portion of glands.

F

Fibromyalgia A chronic pain disorder that affects fibrous connective tissues of the muscles, tendons, and ligaments, and is characterized by the presence of myofascial "tender points." The disorder is often accompanied by fatigue, insomnia, headaches, and/or depression.

Full Sensory Perception The quality of perception that makes use of the physical senses, including touch, hearing, sight, and smell. It is an important factor in developing practical, intuitive skills in clinical practice.

Functionality Individual ability to function in one's body, utilizing the physiological functions of the body in a normal state or in healthy adaptation to changes. Also can refer to mental function, for example, cognitive function and memory.

G

Galvanic skin response A change in the electrical resistance of the skin that is a physiochemical response to a change in emotional state.

Glaucoma A disease of the eye that is characterized by an increase in intraocular pressure, resulting in damage to the optic nerve, leading to blindness. Early stages of the disease present as loss of peripheral vision.

Grief A normal emotional response to an external loss; distinguished from a depressive disorder, since it usually subsides after a reasonable time.

Grounding A state of being in which the individual is confident of one's skills, and carries a sense of stability and connection to the earth. As with a radio, the quality of "grounding into the earth" allows a greater ability to tune into the world around oneself, and still maintain a focus to work and communicate clearly with others.

H

Healing The process of making one well or of restoring to a state of health or wholeness. While curing implies the notion of ridding one of disease, healing emphasizes the acknowledgment of the individual as a whole human being, regardless of one's current condition.

Hepatitis Inflammation of the liver, usually due to viral infection. Various types include A, B, and C.

HIV The human immunodeficiency virus, which attacks the immune system, leaving the victim vulnerable to a host of opportunistic infections. Infection with HIV is the cause of acquired immune deficiency syndrome (AIDS).

Homeostasis The balanced state of all the body's systems and the chemical and neurological processes that control them.

Hospice An institution that provides a centralized program of palliative and supportive services to dying persons and their families, in the form of physical, psychological, social, and spiritual care. Services are provided by an interdisciplinary team of professionals and volunteers who are available to provide care to patients in their homes or in specialized in-patient settings.

Hypoglycemia Abnormally low levels of glucose in the blood.

Hyperglycemia Abnormally high levels of glucose in the blood; a primary sign of diabetes mellitus.

I

Integrative Massage Originally called Neo Reichian Massage, this style of bodywork was influenced by the psychotherapeutic work of Wilhelm Reich, and his theory regarding the relationship of psychological tension to muscular armor in the body. Developed at the Boulder College of Massage Therapy in the 1970s, integrative massage uses strokes derived from Swedish massage to release this muscular armor, thereby creating the experience of relaxation while fostering integration of body, heart, and mind. Broad, fluid strokes, which are applied in a slow rhythm, move from the core of the body to the periphery, while emphasizing the interconnectiveness of the parts of the body.

The term also refers to therapeutic massage that combines eclectic techniques and approaches.

Intuition The process of arriving at a conclusion without having gone through a rational decision making process. It is the sense of knowing what to do without necessarily knowing why. It may be a sudden insight based on perceptions that are primarily unconscious. See **Full Sensory Perception.**

K

Ki Japanese word meaning "vital energy," used to describe the flow of energy or life force throughout the body. Also called **chi** in Chinese.

L

Lipodystrophy Disturbance of fat metabolism, causing uneven distribution of fat in the body. It may involve loss of fat from face, arms, and legs, and accumulation of fat in other areas, such as the back of the neck. There can also be associated high levels of cholesterol and triglycerides.

M

Macronutrients The basic components of food; protein, fat, and carbohydrates.

Macular degeneration A disease of the eye characterized by degeneration of the macula of the retina, resulting in loss of central vision.

Medical massage Any form of massage or bodywork that is practiced with the intention of promoting the health and well-being of the client. Emphasis may be on treatment of a specific condition, or it may be to induce an overall state of relaxation. Also called *therapeutic massage* or *clinical massage.*

Meridian A pathway or channel of energy in the body, used to describe the flow of *chi* or *ki* in the body, according to Asian bodywork traditions of acupuncture and acupressure.

Micronutrients Nutritional components of food other than the macronutrients (protein, fat, carbohydrate); vitamins and minerals.

Motor point Point where the motor nerve enters the muscle, and where visible contraction can be elicited with minimal stimulation.

Multiple sclerosis A disease that involves the destruction of the myelin sheaths around both motor and sensory neurons in the central nervous system, resulting in spasticity of muscles, tremors, fatigue, and progressive loss of motor function. Symptoms of multiple sclerosis can be exacerbating-remitting—meaning that there are episodes of neurologic dysfunction followed by periods of recovery.

Muscle tissue A type of tissue composed of contractile cells; it affects movement of an organ or part of the body.

Muscular dystrophies A group of more than 30 genetic diseases characterized by progressive weakness and degeneration of the skeletal muscles that control movement. Loss of muscle function can also affect the cardiac muscle and the muscles affecting respiratory function.

Myelin A fatty substance that forms an insulating sheath around various nerves in the body. It increases the speed of nerve impulse conduction.

Myopia Defect in vision in which objects can be seen distinctly only when they are very close to the eyes. Also known as nearsightedness.

N

Natural scent therapy The use of natural scents to enhance the quality of life. This therapy avoids the use of artificial chemical scents and concentrated essential oils in favor of scents used in cooking, herbal teas, fresh flowers, and fragrant plants and oils.

Nervous tissue Cells that make up the nervous system—including the brain, spinal cord, and nerves—that are specialized to generate and conduct electrical impulses throughout the body.

Neuropeptide An endogenous peptide (as an endorphin) that influences neural activity or functioning.

Nociceptor A peripheral nerve organ or mechanism for the reception and transmission of painful or injurious stimuli.

Nutrient density Refers to food that is high in nutrient content relative to the number of calories they contain.

O

Orthopedic massage An approach to massage that is designed to assess and treat specific soft-tissue pain or dysfunction. It is used in the treatment of neuromuscular injuries, to enhance athletic performance, or to assist others in physical conditioning.

Osteoarthritis A degenerative condition of the joints, characterized by the destruction of articular cartilage, particularly in weight-bearing joints. Usually due to wear and tear of the joints, and consequent irritation and inflammation, it is a common condition in old age. There may be overgrowth of bone and the formation of bone spurs. It is usually accompanied by mild to severe pain, and involves progressive loss of function.

Oxytocin A hormone produced by the pituitary gland that is involved in uterine contractions in labor, as well as in lactation. It is associated with human bonding behaviors, and is believed to have a role in stress reduction by reducing blood pressure and cortisol levels, and increasing tolerance to pain.

P

Pain An unpleasant sensation associated with actual or potential tissue damage and mediated by specific nerve fibers to the brain, where its conscious appreciation may be modified by various factors.

Pain-Spasm-Pain Cycle A theory proposed by Janet Travell (1942) that states: "Painfulness of the skeletal muscle presumably caused the muscle to spasm, which in turn caused more pain, establishing a self-perpetuating cycle." Techniques of massage can be used to break that cycle.

Palliative Denotes the alleviation of symptoms without curing the underlying cause, to reduce the severity of symptoms, or to comfort the individual suffering with injury or illness.

Parasympathetic nervous system A division of the autonomic nervous system that is concerned with restoration and conservation of body energy.

Parkinson disease A chronic nervous system disease, characterized by a fine, slowly spreading tremor, muscular weakness and rigidity, and irregularities of the gait.

Perception A cognitive awareness derived from sensory stimulus; the mental interpretation or meaning derived from sensory stimulus.

Peripheral neuropathy Damage to the nerves of the hands, arms, feet, or legs resulting in numbness, pain, or weakness; a complication of diabetes and other illnesses.

Post-polio syndrome A variety of musculoskeletal symptoms and muscular atrophy that create new difficulties with activities of daily living 25 to 39 years after the original symptoms caused by the viral infection of poliomyelitis.

Postural sway The subtle rocking motion that occurs when sitting or standing in a still, upright position, caused by the intermittent contractions of the tonic muscles. This involuntary swaying continually rebalances the body around its vertical axis.

Presbyopia A loss of elasticity of the lens of the eye due to advancing age, with resulting inability to focus on near objects.

Prone The position of the body when lying face downward.

R

Retinopathy Pathology of the eye, characterized by damage to the retina of the eye, leading to blindness. Diabetic retinopathy is a form of the disease resulting from long-term complications of diabetes that affect the fine blood vessels of the eye. Can be treated by laser surgery.

Rheumatoid arthritis A chronic autoimmune disease characterized by inflammatory changes in the joints, particularly those of the hands and the feet. Changes in the synovial membranes and other connective tissues can lead to deformities of the joints and consequent dysfunction. It affects people of all ages.

S

Scope of practice Denotes the appropriate guidelines by which a person may practice within their profession or line of work, defining which procedures, techniques and methodologies are allowable and which are excluded by the person's training and certification or licensing.

Senescence The process by which the capacity for cell division, growth, and function is lost over time, ultimately leading to an incompatibility with life—that is, the process of senescence ends in death.

Sensation Physical feeling derived from the operation or function of the sense organs of the body.

Septicemia Systemic disease caused by the spread of microorganisms and their toxins via the circulating blood.

Shiatsu A Japanese style of bodywork based on an awareness of energy pathways or meridians in the body. Pressure is applied on, along, or around the meridians to increase the flow of energy, release tension, and allow deep relaxation. In traditional Shiatsu, the client is usually clothed and lies on a cotton mat called a futon. Shiatsu literally translates as "finger pressure," but other parts of the body, such as thumbs, hands, or feet may be used to apply pressure.

Spasm A sudden involuntary contraction of one or more muscles; includes cramps and contractures. Spasms may be clonic (characterized by alternate contractions and relaxation) or tonic (sustained).

Standard Precautions Standard Precautions are guidelines adopted by the Centers for Disease Control and Prevention that are designed to reduce the risk of transmission of microorganisms from both recognized and unrecognized sources of infection in hospitals and other medical settings. Standard Precautions synthesize the major features of Universal Precautions (blood and body fluid precautions) and body substance isolation (pathogens from moist body surfaces). Standard Precautions apply to blood; all body fluids, secretions, and excretions except sweat, regardless of whether they contain visible blood; non-intact skin; and mucous membranes.

Stroke See **Cerebrovascular accident (CVA)**

Superficial fascia Composed of adipose tissue and loose connective tissue, the superficial fascia is located beneath the skin. Varying in thickness, it covers the entire body, providing insulation and protection for the deep fascia, muscles, and organs beneath it. It stores fat and water and provides passageways for nerves and blood and lymph vessels.

Supine The position of the body when lying face upward.

Swedish massage A commonly practiced form of massage, the intention of which is to promote circulation of blood and lymph and release muscular tension. It uses a variety of strokes, including effleurage (gliding), petrissage (kneading), friction, vibration, tapotement (percussion), and joint movement. It is usually practiced on a client who is lying on a massage table, disrobed but fully draped. The therapist usually uses lotion or oil when performing the massage. See **Conventional massage.**

Sympathetic nervous system A division of the autonomic nervous system, which is involved in the expenditure of energy in the body.

T

Tactile receptor A sensory nerve ending that responds to various kinds of stimulation, like heat, cold, pressure, or pain.

Tendonitis Inflammation of a tendon, the fibrous connective tissue that attaches muscle to bone.

Therapeutic massage Any form of massage or bodywork that is practiced with the intention of promoting the health and well-being of the client. Emphasis may be on treatment of a specific condition, or to induce an overall state of relaxation. Also called **medical massage.**

Tonic points Specific acupressure points in the body known to relieve muscular tension and pain, contribute to relaxation, and promote a sense of well-being. Many of them correspond with the motor points of the muscles.

Transient ischemic attack (TIA) Temporary interference with blood supply to the brain. Symptoms may last a few minutes up to several hours, and there is usually no evidence of permanent brain or neurological damage following the attack. TIAs can be warning signs of impending stroke.

U

Universal Precautions Guidelines set forth by the Centers for Disease Control and Prevention that are observed to protect against blood-borne pathogens. They involve the use of protective barriers such as gloves, gowns, masks, or protective eyewear to reduce the risk of exposure of the healthcare worker's skin or mucous membranes to potentially infectious materials.

V

Vascular dementia A syndrome of intellectual decline caused by changes in the cardiovascular system and diminished blood flow to the brain. In severe cases the loss of mental function is progressive. In some cases it is temporary, and the patient is able to recover function with treatment of the underlying circulatory condition. It can be the result of stroke or transient ischemic attack.

Index

Page numbers in *italics* denote figures; page numbers followed by *t* indicate tables.